Health Research Fundamentals

A Companion to NIeCer 101 Course

First Edition

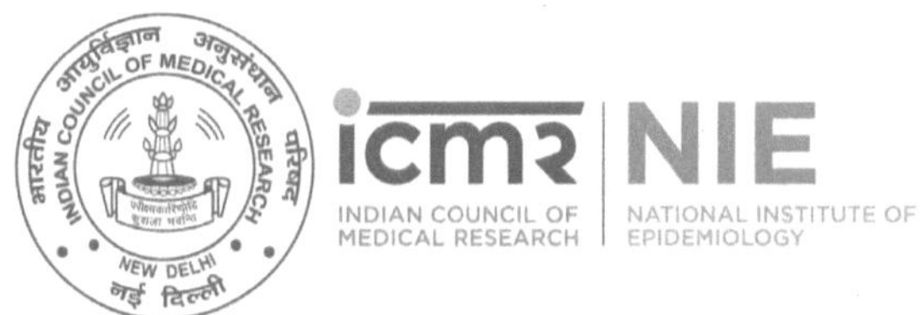

EDITORS

P MANICKAM
BSMS, MSc (Epid), PhD
Scientist F, ICMR - National Institute of Epidemiology

TARUN BHATNAGAR
MD (PSM), PhD (Epid), PGDBE
Scientist F, ICMR - National Institute of Epidemiology

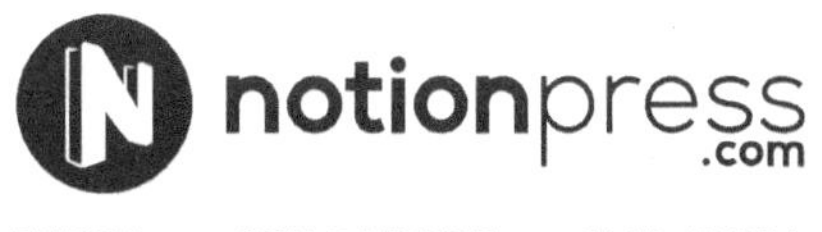

INDIA • SINGAPORE • MALAYSIA

ISBN 979-8-88935-941-8

CONTENTS

SECTION II: EPIDEMIOLOGICAL CONSIDERATIONS IN DESIGNING A RESEARCH STUDY

SECTION III: BIO-STATISTICAL CONSIDERATIONS IN DESIGNING A RESEARCH STUDY

SECTION VI: WRITING A RESEARCH PROTOCOL

APPENDICES

LIST OF FIGURES

LIST OF TABLES

FOREWORD

Dear readers,

I am really happy to inform you that my colleagues from the ICMR-National Institute of Epidemiology (ICMR-NIE) have produced this book titled 'Health Research Fundamentals' as a companion study material to their ongoing online course, NIeCer 101. This book is authored by the scientific faculty of the ICMR School of Public Health at ICMR-NIE. The authors have several years of experience in teaching and research in the field of public health and epidemiology. Besides serving as an aide to the NIeCer 101 online course, this book will be helpful to all those interested in learning about the procedures and principles involved in planning and implementing human health research studies. The contents of this book will also be useful to those who are engaged in capacity building in the area of health research.

I encourage and strongly suggest that all current and future health researchers make use of this book to enhance their knowledge and skills in health research. The MOOC (Massive Open Online Course) offered by NIE would also be a valuable aid to building skills in this area.

I appreciate the erudite editors and the contributors for bringing out this comprehensive book that can really help shape epidemiological research skills in India.

Best wishes,

Soumya Swaminathan,
Former Chief Scientist, World Health Organisation.

PREFACE AND ACKNOWLEDGEMENTS

தொட்டனைத் தூறும் மணற்கேணி மாந்தர்க்குக்
கற்றனைத் தூறும் அறிவு. (திருக்குறள் 396; திருவள்ளுவர்)

In sandy soil, when deep you delve, you reach the springs below;
The more you learn, the freer streams of wisdom flow.

(Thirukural 396; Thiruvalluvar)

Research is the systematic investigation into a specific field of knowledge undertaken to establish a fact or a principle in advancement to existing knowledge. Health research is integral to protecting and promoting health through evidence-based actions. It is the key to identifying individual and community-level health problems and seeking interventions based on scientific investigation and causal reasoning.

The ICMR-NIE team is pleased to present the book, 'Health Research Fundamentals' for your eyes and brains. This book is primarily a by-product of our initiatives towards launching health-related Massive Open Online Courses (MOOCs) in the name of **NI**E-ICMR **e**-**Cer**tificate (NIeCer) courses. In 2016, we designed and started offering our inaugural MOOC, *NIeCer 101: Health Research Fundamentals,* capitalising on the demand and growing niche of online courses in India. We were fortunate enough to partner with India's MOOCs initiative, SWAYAM, which is run by the Ministry of Education. Our foray into the MOOCs world was fully facilitated and supported by the National Programme for Technology Enhanced Learning (NPTEL), which is one of SWAYAM's national coordinators located at IIT Madras in Chennai. Through this attempt, we expect to realise the potential and objective of MOOCs in reaching out to potential researchers, irrespective of qualification, but interested in building their foundations in health research. The NIeCER 101 course is available at https://nie.gov.in/icmr_sph/HRF.html.

While working on the course run, we thought of collating the course materials into a book. Our objective, however, is not to add another book to the potpourri of existing resources available on research methods. Rather, our main aim is to ensure that this book serves as an add-on to the NIeCer101 course. We believe that this book can serve as a primer for audiences who are looking for a theoretical foundation and practical experiences around biomedical and health research methods.

This book has 6 sections and 22 chapters that summarise the principles and practices in epidemiology, biostatistics and research methods. The chapters will help readers to conceptualise, design, plan, propose, conduct and report a research study using epidemiological and biostatistical tools.

The first section of the book discusses ways of conceptualising a research study. This section begins with an overview of the health research process and describes the various dimensions and scope of health research. Subsequently, the components of research questions, the need to formulate a good research question and objectives, the importance of literature review and the skills required to retrieve, interpret and critically appraise scientific literature are dealt with. Section 2 on epidemiological considerations in designing a research study introduces quantitative and qualitative research methods. This section familiarises the readers with the measures that are used to quantify health problems in a population, the types of epidemiological study designs, the interpretation of causal relationships, and the validation of epidemiological studies. Section 3 presents the biostatistical considerations for designing a research study. In this section, the readers are introduced to basic biostatistical techniques that will facilitate them in measuring the study variables and determining the sampling techniques.

Sections 4 and 5 present a step-by-step guide to the processes involved in designing and conducting a research study. These sections will enable readers to apply the theoretical knowledge of fundamental epidemiology and biostatistics to real-life problems and find potential solutions. Section 5 gives an overview of the ethical aspects to be taken into consideration while conducting health research. In the last section, we present ways of developing a concept note and writing a research proposal. This section will provide readers with the templates for the concept paper and research protocol, with an emphasis on the structure and reporting guidelines.

We would like to close this preface by acknowledging the collective efforts of the NIeCer team in producing this book. Many people have contributed enormously to the development of the course contents of this book. The faculty members of the ICMR School of Public Health at ICMR-NIE deserve special mention for giving us their time and valuable contributions in laying out the book's contents. Dr. E. Rajalakshmi and Dr. Malathi Mathiyazhakan took special interest towards the release of the book by reviewing and copy-editing various sections of the book and working closely with the publishers. We sincerely appreciate the team of consultants, the Information Officer, Mr. S. Satish, the IT team and the ICMR-NIE administration for their valuable support throughout this endeavour.

P Manickam

Tarun Bhatnagar

SECTION I

CONCEPTUALISING A RESEARCH STUDY

INTRODUCTION TO HEALTH RESEARCH

Sanjay Mehendale

Learning Objectives

At the end of this chapter, readers will be able to:

1. Describe various dimensions of health research
2. Explain the fundamental principles and key components of the health research process
3. Outline various challenges in designing and implementing research studies

This chapter will give you an overview of health research. Before we pursue any research, it is essential to understand the various dimensions, fundamental principles, processes and scope of such research. Certain critical considerations involved in planning a health research are understanding the focus of health research, finding solutions for the problems identified, identifying approaches to addressing errors and determining study methods and measurements.

1.1 DIMENSIONS OF HEALTH RESEARCH

Health research can be conducted for theoretical purposes, and when some good evidence is generated from it, the researcher can opt for '**Applied Research**'. There are also prevention and therapeutic angles for conducting health research. Emerging preventive technologies as well as newer therapeutic options need to be tested using appropriate research methods. '**Bench-Based Research**' is a type of research in which scientists in white coats work in laboratories with animals like mice and monkeys. The findings of such animal studies have no significance until they are followed up with '**Bedside Research**', wherein they are applied on patients to alleviate or prevent disease. Both bench-based and bedside research are equally significant and must be conducted rigorously. '**Exploratory Research**' is a type of research wherein the investigator does not know much about the context to begin with, and therefore employs various methods to find clues for further research. On the other hand, when previously known information is strengthened or when we gather additional new information that could be of practical value, it is called '**Confirmatory Research**'.

'**Implementation Research**' and '**Translational Research**' have recently gained wide attention. In India, several national health programmes have been launched periodically to address maternal and child health, nutrition, communicable and non-communicable diseases and strengthening of the health system. **Implementation research** focuses on understanding whether such programmes are working as per plan after launch. Information collected in such research can aid mid-course corrections and help policymakers decide whether these programmes are necessary in the first place. If deemed necessary, it helps identify specific programme areas that need strengthening. **Translational research** is the adaptation of bench-based research from laboratories to patient bedside, which involves technological developments for human benefit and welfare.

1.2 FUNDAMENTAL PRINCIPLES IN HEALTH RESEARCH

We have to bear in mind some important principles while conducting health research. First, the researcher has to plan adequately before conducting the research. The planning stage is critical, and if enough time is not spent or subject matter experts not involved at this stage, a novice researcher is likely to overlook issues that could have been avoided during research implementation. Second, the researcher must involve a multidisciplinary team of members who have expertise in the relevant field of study, as independent, single-handed researches succeed very rarely.

Third, prior to implementing the research, the research proposal has to undergo several levels of review. The reviews can be scientific, ethical or regulatory in nature. **Scientific reviews** inspect the novelty of the concept, and the rationality and justification for conducting the said research. It is also vital to understand the rationale for conducting a study in a specific country, pertaining to the local context. **Ethics review** focuses on determining whether the participants are adequately protected during the process of the research.

People who willingly participate in a research are called human participants or participants. Ethics review ensures that the development and advances attributed to the research are not happening at the cost of human participants. Researchers should not do anything that can harm the participants in the short or long run.

In addition, there are certain in-country procedures or in-country reviews called **regulatory reviews**. In these reviews, the reviewers scrutinise any foreign funding received for the intended research, and whether sample shipments and data sharing are involved. In India, data sharing is considered as sharing of one's intellectual property; hence, the regulatory authorities ensure that the researcher's intellectual properties are adequately protected. Some projects may involve the exchange of visitors, which are reviewed mandatorily by regulatory committees. Several countries have set rules and regulations regarding the exchange of visitors in research projects.

1.3 PROCESS OF HEALTH RESEARCH

Health research in itself is a process. It involves multiple tasks, with every one of them given due importance. Data collection is one such task that is conducted for a specific purpose. Researchers must use appropriate data collection instruments to maintain data quality. Only then can they draw meaningful conclusions and take appropriate decisions. These decisions can assist policymakers and program managers in deciding whether to translate learning from the research into appropriate action for the prevention and control of diseases. Such action can be taken at an individual level or at a mass level. This action that is based on generated evidence is called **evidence-based action**. The primary purpose of this method of action is to ensure a reduction in suffering and, ultimately, an improvement in the health and well-being of a specific population or community.

1.4 BREADTH AND DEPTH OF INQUIRY IN HEALTH RESEARCH

The information that we collect in research can have a wide array in terms of breadth and depth of inquiry. For example, when we collect data from human participants regarding host characteristics, they can be healthy, susceptible to disease, diseased or dead due to that particular disease. We have to decide on appropriate ways to collect the required information from these diverse participants. A disease cannot occur unless there are other contributing factors in an individual; these factors form the multifactorial origin for the occurrence of the disease. It is well established that the surrounding environment and society in which we live play a very significant role in the occurrence of diseases. Environmental factors like climate, housing, vectors and animals in the vicinity and social factors such as socio-cultural practices in the community and family structure not only affect the physical and mental health of individuals but also result in the occurrence of disease. Information about such factors can be collected during the data collection stage.

Another important dimension in health research is healthcare infrastructure. Timely access to health care and its delivery are critical factors related to health and disease. Studies have shown that complications and death rates are high among people with poor healthcare access.

Therefore, each problem must be looked at from multiple angles, and inclusive data needs to be collected. These factors about which data are collected are called study variables. It is crucial to capture accurate information on these study variables when conducting health research.

1.5 BROAD SCOPE OF HEALTH RESEARCH

The scope of health research ranges from collecting additional or new information, and verifying and confirming available information, to explaining cause and effect relationships. Largely, when we think of research, we think about discovering new information. However, research could either generate new information or, at times, find additional information to supplement existing information.

1.5.1 Additional Information

Take for example, the following research question: "Are more diphtheria and pertussis cases reported among adults in recent times?"

It is well established that diphtheria and pertussis are diseases that affect children. However, recently there have been some rare instances of their occurrence in adults. So, we need to figure out why and where this is happening, which can provide additional information to the existing literature.

1.5.2 New Information

On the other hand, some researchers may also conduct research to find new information.

For example, consider the following research question: "What are the differences in the full genome structure of Hepatitis 'B' and Hepatitis 'E' viruses?"

This question could imply deriving an understanding of the pathogenic impact of the viruses on human beings. It could also play a significant role in aiding the decision-making process with respect to the development of a vaccine against those viruses and reveal a dimension unknown so far.

1.5.3 Verifying and Confirming Available Information

Another objective that one can pursue in health research is verifying and confirming available information. In recent times, most research in our country has been focused on this.

For example, it is well known that the food habits of people have changed rapidly in the last two decades, with more people shifting towards pre-cooked or packaged food as compared to home-cooked fresh meals. A researcher can use health research to find out whether pre-cooked or packaged food increases the number of cases and complications of diabetes mellitus.

The research question, in this case, can be: "Is there an increase in the incidence and complication of diabetes mellitus with increased consumption of pre-cooked or packaged food?"

1.5.4 Cause and Effect Relationship

Health research can also focus on finding cause-and-effect relationships that can be applied in multiple situations.

For example, a researcher wants to know,

"Does the presence of a particular co-receptor (cause) on CD4 cells protect against HIV infection (effect)?"

A specific co-receptor is present in a type of white blood cells called CD4 cells in the human body. These are supposed to protect against HIV infection. This research will evaluate whether there is a cause-and-effect relationship between the presence of co-receptors on the CD4 cells and protection from HIV infection.

Let us look at another example: "Are breast cancers more common in breast implant recipients?"

Breast implant operations are being conducted increasingly in recent times. Here, the researcher wants to know if breast implant (cause) recipients are more likely to develop breast cancer (effect).

1.5.5 Testing of New Interventions

Another important area in health research is testing new interventions like new drugs, new vaccines or new tools for the prevention, treatment and control of a disease.

For example, tuberculosis is one of the most common opportunistic infections among HIV-infected individuals, which may turn out to be fatal eventually. Isoniazid is a potent drug that is used to treat tuberculosis. A researcher wants to know,

"Can isoniazid prophylaxis delay the onset of tuberculosis in HIV-infected persons?"

This is an important intervention that could reduce mortality associated with HIV by preventing the occurrence of tuberculosis in HIV-infected persons.

Let us look at another example. Indoor air pollution has gained much attention recently, particularly in rural areas. So, a researcher wants to find out,

"Will the introduction of smokeless stoves reduce respiratory morbidity and mortality in rural areas?"

Here, the introduction of smokeless stoves in rural areas is the intervention that may or may not reduce respiratory illness-related morbidity and mortality, which is the outcome of interest.

1.5.6 Evaluation of Programmes

The government runs various ongoing public health programmes that are vertical in nature, focusing on a particular disease or a group of diseases. In India, general health services are provided by state-level health centres, while national-level health programmes are operated and funded by the Central Government. These programmes have to be assessed to determine whether the standard operating procedures were followed and whether the programmes had an impact on improving outcomes.

For example, according to the National Family Health Survey-4, 50% of pregnant women in India have anaemia. Anaemia, when not treated, can lead to severe complications and adverse perinatal outcomes. Under the Intensified National Iron Plus Initiative, injectable iron sucrose is made available to women in addition to oral iron supplementation to help improve their haemoglobin level during pregnancy. A researcher wants to know,

"Whether additional injectable iron sucrose is a better alternative to treat pregnancy-related anaemia when compared to oral iron alone."

Evaluation of this programme can, therefore, improve outcomes of pregnancy, help to check the feasibility of implementing the intervention and help prioritise the allocation of funds.

Let us look at another example:

"Will the Integrated Disease Programme be able to predict epidemics of influenza and bird flu in India?"

Integrated Disease Surveillance Programme (IDSP) is an important flagship programme of the Government of India to combat communicable diseases. Here, the researcher wants to assess whether newer and emerging diseases like H1N1 and bird flu can be predicted using data collected through IDSP, so that preventive and control measures could be taken on time.

1.6 CHOOSING THE RIGHT STUDY DESIGN

Choosing the right study design is crucial for sound research. Misjudgements can lead to futile research and an incomplete understanding of the problem in question. Broadly, study designs can be quantitative or qualitative. **Quantitative studies** include objective measurements and numerical representation of the problem under study. They include data collection using structured questionnaires with pre-specified options based on existing knowledge. On the other hand, **qualitative studies** are subjective and used to understand perceptions and gain insight into a problem. Observations, free listing, group discussions and interviews are a few methods employed in qualitative research. Topic guides or interview guides with open-ended questions and probes are employed to collect data in qualitative research.

Studies can also be classified as observational or experimental. In epidemiological terms, **observational studies** are those in which the investigators merely observe and do not change the environment of the study participants. On the other hand, in **experimental studies**, the investigator manipulates the environment by introducing a new intervention or withdrawing an existing element. Manipulation of the environment is the key differentiating feature between these two studies.

Depending on the direction of inquiry, studies can be classified as retrospective or prospective. In **retrospective studies**, information on the outcome that is being studied is already available. We go back in time to ascertain whether individuals with a particular outcome were exposed to a risk factor or not. On the contrary, in a **prospective study**, we begin with people at risk or susceptible to a particular disease. The outcome occurs in the future. We work with a control group or comparison group. Both these groups are monitored to assess how many people who were disease-free at the beginning of the study developed the disease in question.

1.7 KEY CONSIDERATIONS FOR THE PLANNING PHASE

Planning is the crux of research. Research involves investment in terms of money, manpower and time. Hence, there should be adequate rationale or justification for conducting research. The original research question should be clear and focused on providing adequate justification. In addition, the case definitions of study variables and outcomes should be standard and unambiguous. For example, if a researcher wants to study carcinoma cervix, then the clear delineation of what is considered carcinoma in situ and invasive carcinoma must be known to everybody involved in that particular research.

Other critical aspects include how we draw a sample from the population and how we determine the sample size for the study. The sample should be representative of the population that is being studied. This will ensure 'external validity' or 'generalisability', which means extrapolating the findings of a study based on a sample to the population from which the sample was drawn. Adequate sample size is yet another requisite for a powerful study that helps to draw meaningful inferences.

1.8 ERROR PREDICTION AND MINIMALISATION

Despite meticulous planning, research can never be completely free from errors. However, we can predict and minimise them by choosing an appropriate study design. Errors can be of two types—random errors and systematic errors. Random errors occur due to variability by chance. Suppose a researcher plans to measure the height of the first five students in a classroom of 50 students. The mean height drawn from the sample of five students would be different from the actual mean height of all the students in the classroom. This difference in the measurement due to sampling that has occurred by chance is called a **random error**. Random errors cannot be completely eliminated from research studies. However, we can minimise them by increasing the sample size. A large sample size will minimise inter-individual variation within the sample.

Systematic error or bias occurs as a result of faulty procedures or inconsistencies in measurements. It may occur due to dissimilarities in participant recruitment, differences in the data collection method or measurement errors. Systematic errors can be minimised by improving the study design.

1.9 CHALLENGES IN DESIGN AND IMPLEMENTATION

A thorough literature review can aid the researcher in addressing potential issues in designing and implementing the research. It will give researchers an idea about two important factors: confounders and effect modifiers that affect the results of their research.

A **confounder** is an independent variable other than the study variable that affects both the study variable as well as the outcome. The concept of confounders is explained with examples in Chapter 8: Validity of Epidemiological Studies. If researchers do not recruit participants with confounding characteristics, they might end up with very few participants. Therefore, it is crucial to identify confounders and collect information on all known confounders. This can be done at the statistical analysis phase of the study. On the other hand, **effect modifiers** can alter or distort the true relationship between the study variable and the outcome by altering the effect of the study variable on the outcome. A thorough literature search must be done to identify the kind of effect that effect modifiers are likely to have on the outcome variable. One strategy is to not include people with effect modifiers in the study.

1.10 MAJOR ISSUES IN STUDY METHODS AND MEASUREMENTS

Research can have multiple stages. A pilot study is a research conducted on a small scale to understand the challenges the researcher is likely to face during data collection, carrying out research procedures, conducting interviews, getting informed consent and determining the feasibility and acceptability of the study.

While selecting the study population, the inclusion and exclusion criteria should be clearly stated to ensure the recruitment of eligible participants only. The recruitment targets and specific strategies to be used for recruiting should be clearly spelt out in the standard operating procedures. Depending on the research question, the study setting, which is the community or the facility from which the participants will be recruited, has to be decided *a priori*.

Data collection instruments must be designed carefully. Poor designing of data collection instruments will lead to inadequate information, which can cause difficulties in drawing meaningful inferences at a later stage. Hence, selecting or designing the appropriate data collection tool is very important.

Health research may sometimes include measuring biochemical parameters using laboratory methods or assays, or other tools. These methods should be standardised and have appropriate internal and external controls (positive and negative controls to ensure quality). The lab should preferably have an external quality assurance program that ensures quality control at all levels. Another focal component is drawing a plan for statistical analysis of the study upfront. This will give the researcher a clear idea of how to collect the data and what the results of the study will look like eventually.

1.11 FOCUS OF HEALTH RESEARCH

Before conducting health research, researchers need to orient themselves towards what they intend to do. For example, they have to decide whether they want to promote a certain behaviour, promote health, prevent disease or prevent mortality. Some questions that researchers have to keep in mind while conducting health research are:

- "How can the health of the population be improved?"
- "How can we predict the occurrence of disease in an individual?"
- "How can various diseases be prevented?"
- "How can we effectively cure the diseases and reduce the associated morbidity and mortality?"
- "What are various societal, community-based and programmatic interventions for disease prevention and control?"

These are some of the core directions in which health research should be conducted.

1.12 HEALTH RESEARCH FOR PRACTICAL SOLUTIONS

Health research aims to find answers or practical solutions for problems at individual and community levels. At the individual level, promoting healthy behaviour, disease prevention, early diagnosis, prompt treatment and rehabilitation are aspects in the limelight of health research. At the community level, improving community behaviour and practices, implementing prevention and control programmes, supporting affected people and addressing stigma reduction are some focus areas. Investing in health research helps achieve healthy population and healthy nations!

References and Further Reading

1. Chapter 1 - Introduction to research. In: World Health Organization. *Health research methodology: a guide for training in research methods.* Manila: WHO Regional Office for the Western Pacific; 2001: p.1-10. https://apps.who.int/iris/handle/10665/206929
2. Bonita R, Beaglehole R, Kjellstrom T. Chapter 11 - First steps in practical epidemiology. In: 2nd ed. *Basic epidemiology.* Geneva: World Health Organization; 2006: p. 177-87. http://apps.who.int/iris/bitstream/10665/43541/1/9241547073

FORMULATING RESEARCH QUESTION, HYPOTHESIS AND OBJECTIVES

P. Manickam

Learning Objectives

At the end of this chapter, readers will be able to:

1. Paraphrase a research question
2. Distinguish between descriptive and analytical questions
3. Formulate research hypothesis/es
4. Define research objective(s)

The goal of health research is to establish facts or principles through careful and systematic investigation in the area of research. The objective of such an investigation is to improve the health of the population. The first step in the research process is formulating the research question. This chapter covers three areas—(a) spelling out a research question, (b) stating the research hypothesis and (c) formulating the study objectives.

2.1 THE LIFE CYCLE OF RESEARCH

Any research has a life cycle, as shown in Figure 2.1. It begins with an 'uncertainty' or a 'need'. This need is translated into a research question and as study objectives subsequently, and a plan of analysis is formulated to guide the development of the data collection instruments. Using these tools, data are collected and analysed as per the plan, objectives and conclusions are drawn, and recommendations are formulated. Finally, the recommendations are shared with the relevant stakeholders. This process can end with another uncertainty that may begin the cycle for a new research. Therefore, we need to start with a good research question.

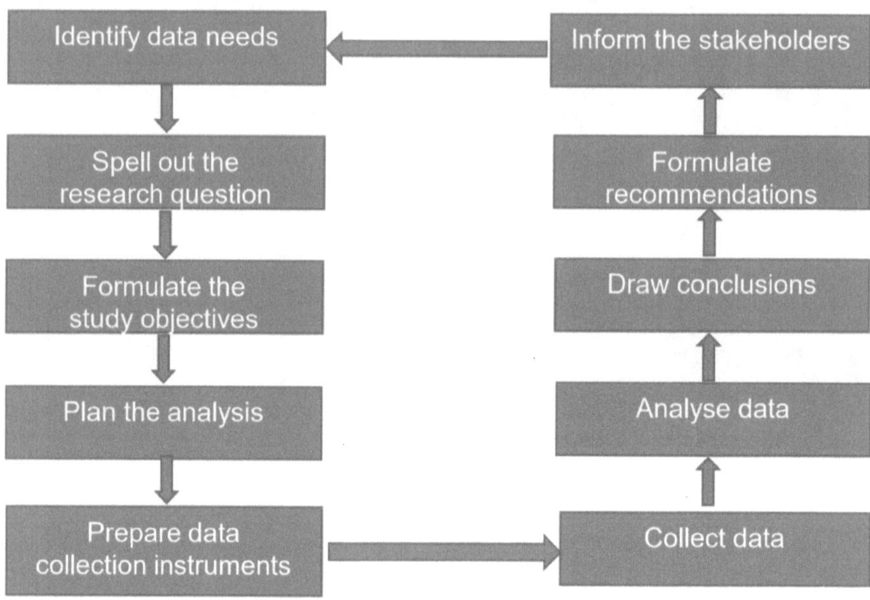

▲ **Figure 2.1:** Life cycle of research

2.2 WHAT IS A RESEARCH QUESTION?

A research question is an uncertainty about something in the population that the researcher wants to resolve by making measurements in the study population. An uncertainty is called 'data needs' in the life cycle of research. We need a clear question to facilitate choosing an optimal study design, identifying the participants to be included, defining the outcomes to be measured and determining the time of measuring the outcomes. A research question is all about refining your ideas into a systematic process of framing a question. It begins with general uncertainty about a health issue, which is then narrowed down into a concrete researchable topic.

2.2.1 Translating Uncertainty Into a Research Question

While translating uncertainty into a research question, we must frame the problem in specific terms. In health research, it could be in clinical or public health terms. The research question must focus on one issue at a time and must be written in simple language so that everybody understands the question. You may choose to use more than one operational verb if required. It must be stated as a question and should link the question, if answered, to what action has to be taken. The research question must state clearly what the researcher wants to know and not what they may want to do or what the study results might ultimately contribute to.

2.3 SOURCES FOR RESEARCH QUESTIONS

There are many sources from which research questions or ideas can be identified. The first source is **literature search** in the area of research interest. Up-to-date information from literature will help generate strong research questions. The second source is **new ideas and techniques**, which can be collected by attending **research meetings** or **conferences**, or in **peer group discussions**, when having a sceptical attitude about the prevailing beliefs and applying new technologies to old issues. The third source is careful **observation** of one's area of work. The fourth source is **in-depth knowledge** about the topic. The last source is a **guide** or a mentor who can help in identifying and framing research questions.

2.4 TYPES OF RESEARCH QUESTIONS

There are two categories of research questions—descriptive research questions and analytical research questions. The research question for any study should fall into either of these categories.

A **descriptive research question** involves observations made to measure a quantity. The quantity could be blood pressure, level of knowledge or extent of a problem in a community such as the burden of a disease. Intervention or comparison groups are not used when conducting research on a descriptive research question. On the contrary, research on an **analytical research question** will involve a comparison group, or could involve an intervention or experiment to test a specific hypothesis.

Example 1: "What is the average level of blood pressure among diabetic patients?" This research question intends to estimate the blood sugar level of people with diabetes. This is an example of a descriptive research question.

Example 2: "Do diabetics have a higher blood pressure than non-diabetic people?" This research question intends to test a hypothesis that blood pressure among diabetic patients is higher than among non-diabetics. This is an analytical research question.

2.5 STEPS IN FRAMING A RESEARCH QUESTION

Figure 2.2 shows the six steps involved in framing a research question.

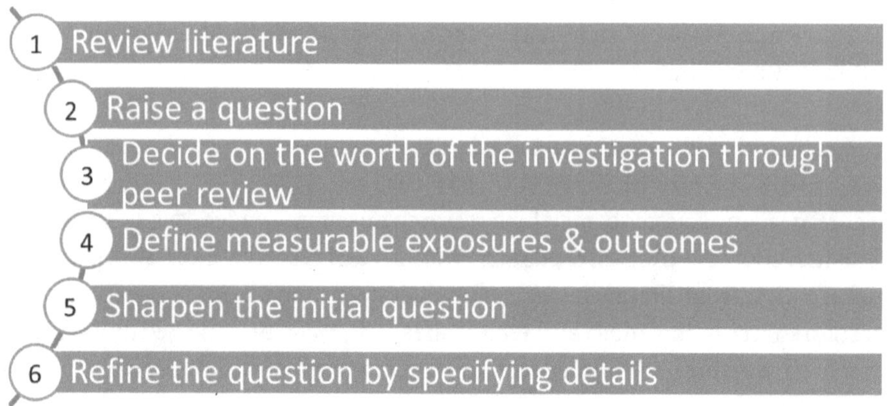

▲ **Figure 2.2:** Steps in framing a research question

Let us take the example of the following research question: "Should diabetics exercise daily?"

The first step is to review literature about the effect of exercise on the human body. Literature shows that exercise reduces blood sugar levels and body fat. It also indicates that exercise provides protection against developing complications due to diabetes. So, the question is worth investigating.

The second step is to modify the research question based on the review of literature. "Can exercise help control blood sugar levels?" This sounds better than the earlier question, but it is still vague. The question needs to be refined. The researcher must define what they mean by exercise and blood sugar level.

The third step is to talk to people/peer groups and investigators with expertise in specialised areas to gain more insight into the topic. What is meant by blood sugar? Is it measured in a fasting, random or post-prandial state? What is the expected level of reduction in blood sugar? Which of the three types of blood sugar gets reduced? Looking through literature might help you come up with more questions about exercise. What is the optimal type of exercise? What is the frequency, intensity and duration of such exercise? Are there any risks for diabetics who engage in exercise? Are there other benefits for diabetics other than a possible reduction in blood sugar?

The fourth step is to define the exposure and outcome. For the purpose of the current example, exercise could be defined as a pre-determined physical activity comprising any body movement produced by skeletal muscles, resulting in an increase in energy expenditure, with the completion of at least one session of 60 minutes every day for one year. You can be more specific about the exercise or physical activity by mentioning the type of exercise, such as walking, jogging, cycling, aerobics or even dancing. The outcome is fasting blood sugar level, which means blood sugar level taken after eight hours of being on an empty stomach.

The fifth step is to sharpen the initial question through the steps mentioned above. In our example, the sharpened question could be, "Does physical activity of one hour a day help reduce fasting blood sugar levels in diabetics?" This question can be further refined by specifying more details. The study population, operational definitions of exposure and outcome, and study design are some factors that can be specified.

For instance, a descriptive question could be, "What is the extent of regular walking that can be undertaken by diabetic (type 2 diabetes) patients?" An analytical question could be, "Does brisk walking by diabetics (type 2 diabetes) for at least one hour a day reduce fasting blood sugar level when compared to those who do not?"

2.6 CRITERIA FOR A RESEARCH QUESTION

After framing a research question, we need to test this question using a 'so what?' test. This test comprises five elements, which are represented using the acronym, '**FINER**'.

F - Is this research question 'feasible' to answer?
I - Is it 'interesting' to answer?
N - Is it 'novel'?
E - Is it 'ethical' to conduct studies about the research question?
R - Is it 'relevant'?

- **Feasibility**: Will the researcher get adequate study participants? Does the researcher have the technical expertise to conduct the study? Does the researcher have the materials and human resources to conduct the study?
- **Interesting**: Are people enthused to engage in this research? Is it worth conducting?
- **Novelty**: Does the research confirm, refute or extend previous findings or provide new information?

- **Ethical**: Based on the research questions, is the research allowable under ethical norms? Will an ethics committee pass this research based on the questions?
- **Relevant**: Is the research relevant in terms of advancing science, advancing practice or influencing policy?

2.7 RESEARCH HYPOTHESIS

A hypothesis is a version of the research question that summarises the study's main elements that establish the basis for statistical tests of significance. It is mainly stated for statistical purposes. The main elements of a hypothesis are 'sample', 'exposures' and 'outcomes'.

Only analytical research questions that involve comparison groups require a statement of hypothesis. An analytical question contains terms such as greater or lesser than, causes, leads to, compared with, more likely than, associated with, related to, similar to, correlated with, and so on. A research question containing any of these terms is an analytical question that requires a hypothesis statement. Purely descriptive questions do not require a statement of hypothesis.

2.8 EXAMPLE OF A RESEARCH HYPOTHESIS

Here is a research hypothesis for the sample research question related to diabetes and exercise, which was discussed earlier:

"In a particular study area, diabetics who engage in brisk walking for at least one hour daily experience an average reduction of 10 mg of fasting blood sugar level compared to those who do not."

The specification of the reduction in fasting blood sugar levels, the study area, and the group of study participants will help the researcher consolidate ideas into statements of null and alternative hypotheses. Thus, the research hypothesis helps to specify certain details in the context of statistical tests and sample size.

2.9 CHARACTERISTICS OF A GOOD RESEARCH HYPOTHESIS

What is a good hypothesis? A good hypothesis should be '**simple**', '**specific**' and '**stated in advance**'. Simple means that there should be one 'exposure' and one 'outcome'. Specific means that there should be no ambiguity about the study variables or study participants. The hypothesis should be stated in advance—'*a priori*'. It should not be discovered at a later stage of the study.

The hypothesis should be focused on the primary objective.

2.10 TRANSLATING RESEARCH QUESTIONS TO OBJECTIVES

Compared to the research question, a statement of objective is stated in scientific and epidemiological terms. It takes the research question in only a few limited axes. It is written in scientific and epidemiological language. There should ideally be no more than one operational verb for each research question. It is ideal to sort objectives as primary and secondary objectives. Each objective should spell out whether it is answering a descriptive question or an analytical or experimental question.

2.11 OBJECTIVES FOR DESCRIPTIVE VS. ANALYTICAL STUDIES

As mentioned earlier, an objective could be a **descriptive objective** or an **analytical objective.** The statement of objectives should be written in scientific and epidemiological terms. It is recommended that it uses the terms that denote the descriptive and analytical nature of the study. In a descriptive study in which we estimate a quantity through observation, the verb '**estimate**' is preferred. For example, "to estimate the prevalence of physical activity in diabetics"—is a **descriptive objective**.

An analytical study should use the terms that denote comparison and state the testing hypothesis in verb form. For example, the verb '**determine**' may be preferred. In the diabetes and exercise example that we have been studying so far, the objective is to determine whether exercise reduces blood sugar levels. Wise choice of the verb is extremely important, and therefore we do not recommend the use of vague words, such as 'to study', in the statement of objectives.

Primary Objective

Recall the research question stated earlier. "Does brisk walking by diabetics (type 2 diabetes) for at least one hour a day reduce fasting blood sugar level compared to those who do not?"

This can be translated into a **primary objective**: "To determine the effect of brisk walking for at least one hour a day on fasting blood sugar level of patients with type 2 diabetes compared to those who do not." Here, the verb 'determine' is appropriate, especially for an analytical objective.

2.12 EXAMPLES OF STUDY OBJECTIVES

Below are some good and bad examples of study objectives.

- "Determine the importance of sedentary lifestyle among diabetics."
  The verb 'determine' is not particularly suited for this statement of objective because it seems to be a descriptive study. Therefore, "Estimate the prevalence of physical activity among diabetics" would be a better way to frame this statement of objective.
- "Assess physical activity and diabetic complications."
  This objective is supposed to address a descriptive study. Therefore, "Estimate the prevalence of physical activity among diabetics" would be a better choice of words. So, the verb 'estimate' is preferable.
- "Evaluate depression and diabetes."
  If this is an analytical study, it may be preferable to use the verb 'determine' rather than 'evaluate'—"Determine whether depression is more common among diabetics than healthy individuals."

Asking the right question can help in finding the right answer. Researchers may answer a research question easily, but then the answer may be of no use. If the research question is poorly framed, try to reframe it,. If the research question is wrong, no amount of hard work will benefit the intention of the researcher. If the research question is correct, the researchers will have an opportunity to do a good job.

References and Further Reading

1. Ratan SK, Anand T, Ratan J. Formulation of research question - stepwise approach. J Indian AssocPediatr Surg. 2019;24(1):15-20.
2. Fandino W. Formulating a good research question: Pearls and pitfalls. Indian J Anaesth. 2019; 63(8):611-6.
3. Chapter 3 - Developing research aims and objectives. In: Thomas DR, Hodges I. Designing and planning your research project: Core skills for social and health researchers. Sage Publications 2010.
4. Hulley SB, Cummings SR. Conceiving the research question. In: Hulley SB, Cummings SR, Browner WS, Grady D, Hearst N, Newman TB, editors. Designing Clinical Research. 4th ed. Philadelphia: Williams & Wilkins; 2013. p. 17-19.

CHAPTER 03

LITERATURE REVIEW

P. Ganesh Kumar

Learning Objectives

At the end of this chapter, readers will be able to:

1. Recognise the importance of performing a literature review
2. Describe the steps involved in performing a literature search
3. Outline the steps of writing a literature review

Literature review is an important process in health research; it is a systematic investigation that is done to increase or revise our existing knowledge about the subject of interest. Research may be basic or applied. **Basic research** involves enhancing existing knowledge, whereas **applied research** involves applying basic research knowledge to develop new knowledge, new processes and new products to identify solutions to a problem. In this context, literature review is an important step in any health research, as it enlightens us about the existing knowledge on the concerned subject.

This chapter describes literature review, how it is performed, the steps involved in literature review and certain ethical concerns in literature review.

3.1 WHY PERFORM A LITERATURE REVIEW?

Research is an important link between what is known and what is unknown. Literature review saves a lot of the researcher's time by retrieving existing knowledge about the concerned subject. For example, if a researcher wants to study physical activity, they need a questionnaire to measure the level of physical activity. When searching relevant studies in literature, they may find an existing questionnaire for physical activity, which they can reuse/repurpose for their research. Literature review also helps to understand the subject matter better and identify potential new research topics and questions. For example, when reading an existing article, a researcher may find certain lacunae or gaps in the existing knowledge, which may inspire them to initiate a new research. Finally, literature review can aid researchers to develop new research methods for an existing subject.

3.2 LITERATURE REVIEW—NOT JUST A SUMMARY

During literature review, the researcher will collect known information about the concerned topic and summarise it as existing evidence. Now, one question may arise in your mind: Is literature review just a summary?

No, literature review is not just a summary. It is primarily information seeking. It involves scanning the literature efficiently using manual or computerised methods to identify potentially useful articles and books. During literature review, the researcher retrieves information on an existing topic from any available resource; it may be a textbook, a manuscript, a published article, or a conference proceeding. After collecting all the relevant literature, the researcher needs to critically appraise the literature and identify useful information about the concerned subject by applying the principles of analyses. Critical appraisal of literature is the most important step in literature review.

3.3 STEPS INVOLVED IN LITERATURE REVIEW

Literature review is a systematic process of organising information and synthesising the results of available evidence. Figure 3.1 provides a diagrammatic representation of the steps involved in literature review.

First, we need to organise the collected information and relate it to the concerned research question. Second, we need to synthesise the available results of the literature and summarise them. This is also called synthesising of results. Third, we need to identify the lacunae in the existing literature. When doing this, we can identify new areas of research. The fourth and final step is to develop a research question for further research.

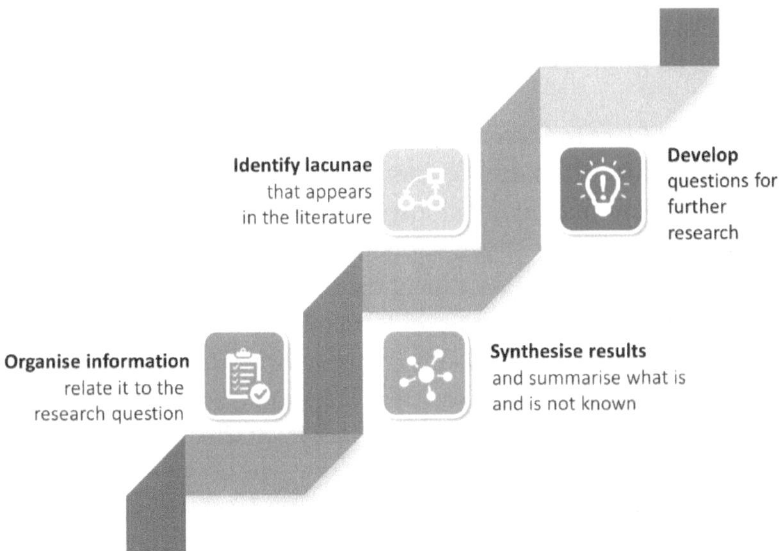

▲ **Figure 3.1:** Steps of literature review

3.4 MECHANISM OF INFORMATION RETRIEVAL IN LITERATURE REVIEW

Various information retrieval mechanisms are available to facilitate the literature review process. Information retrieval tools help in identifying documents that are relevant to the researcher's needs from a large database using a query. A database is a huge collection of information, articles and conference proceedings that are archived, collected or stored. A query is user-defined and usually depends on the research question.

3.4.1 Database Structure and Management

Databases are extensive collections of information and scientific knowledge stored mostly in electronic form. Some books, printed journals and conference proceedings may also be stored in databases. Database management system is a tool that facilitates researchers to retrieve relevant data efficiently from a database. Like the index of a textbook, the database management system maintains a certain mechanism to help researchers retrieve the relevant literature from databases for their research study. This process is called indexing. Researchers collect the required information from a database using a set of queries. This set of queries is what the researcher must define to retrieve the required information from huge databases.

For example, an e-library is an online database of a collection of citations, books, journals, etc., which can be accessed through a computer.

3.4.2 Appropriate Place to Search

Now the question is, where to search for literature? Literature search can be done to retrieve general information about a specific health-related event, disease or research study. In the case of general information, Google is an extensive search engine that has a huge collection of data and facts. Another example is "Health on the Net", which is a non-profit organisation that helps readers to gather reliable information about health-related events. This organisation has an accreditation mechanism for transparent literature search. The Health on the Net certified websites are accredited websites from which researchers can get authorised information.

Professionals and researchers use scientific databases such as PubMed to conduct specific and detailed searches. PubMed is a huge database consisting of over 30 million scientific and bio-medical citations. Scopus is another database that has an immense collection of citations and abstracts of literature. Google Scholar is another portal that stores a large collection of abstracts and articles. Archived full-text articles are usually available in free open-access directories of journals or fee-based e-libraries.

Finally, the researcher may want to refer to or review evidence-based articles. The highest level of evidence that are currently available are systematic review and meta-analysis. Cochrane Library is a database from which researchers can access literature related to systematic review and meta-analysis.

3.5 SEARCHING A DATABASE

Now, let us see how to perform a basic search in a database. To conduct a basic search, we use a Boolean query. This is common in any search engine, such as Google and PubMed. Boolean query is a standardised query that uses operators like AND, OR and NOT. These operators combine keywords or phrases in search engines to conduct basic searches.

For example, we can search for two separate keywords like 'Lung' and 'Infections' here. If we search these two keywords separately, the search engine will return all articles on lungs and infections.

However, we will get different results if these keywords are combined using a Boolean operator, such as 'AND', 'OR' or 'NOT'. When the 'AND' operator is used, as in 'Lung AND Infections', the search engine will retrieve only those articles that include both the keywords, 'Lung' and 'Infections'. If the researcher uses the 'OR' operator, as in 'Lung OR Infections', the search engine will retrieve all the articles that have either of the keywords. Therefore, the researcher will get a large number of search results for this query.

However, if the researcher uses the 'NOT' operator, as in 'Lung NOT Infections', the search engine will remove all information related to 'Infections' from the combined search results. Therefore, it will return only those articles that contain the keyword 'Lung' but not 'Infections'.

3.5.1 PubMed

PubMed has the most popular and widespread collection of biomedical and scientific literature. It comprises more than 30 million citations of biomedical literature. PubMed was created and is maintained by the National Center for Biotechnology Information (NCBI) at the US National Library of Medicine (NLM), situated at the National Institutes of Health (NIH). This is a free and open-access database from which researchers can easily get citations and abstracts related to biomedicine, life sciences and other related fields of study. PubMed does not contain full-text articles; however, it provides links to full-text articles whenever available. Each abstract contains links to the resource where the full-text article is available in PubMed Central (PMC) or the publisher's website. PMC is a part of PubMed that archives the full text of articles.

The US NLM maintains its own set of pre-defined vocabulary terms, called Medical Subject Headings (MeSH). The MeSH thesaurus is a controlled and hierarchically-arranged vocabulary. 'Keywords' are listed below the abstract section of each journal article. If the keywords of an article are in concordance with the NLM-defined vocabulary or MeSH, then that article will have a higher chance of getting identified by a set of systematic query mechanisms. Therefore, MeSH terminologies are extremely important for retrieving literature. Researchers can access the entire MeSH database from the PubMed webpage.

On the PubMed portal, video tutorials are made available for researchers. These tutorials explain how to search PubMed, how to search using a MeSH terminology, how to search using a single citation manager and how to use additional filters like author, study designs, etc.

3.6 SEARCHING IN PUBMED USING A BOOLEAN QUERY

The search results of a basic search query using a Boolean inquiry in PubMed are shown in Figure 3.2 below. This is the kind of results that a researcher will get when performing a basic search on PubMed.

Observe the screenshots in Figure 3.2 below. When a Boolean inquiry is made for the keyword 'Lung', the database retrieves a total of 911,718 items. Whereas, when only the keyword 'Infections' is searched, the total number of items retrieved is 3,418,699.

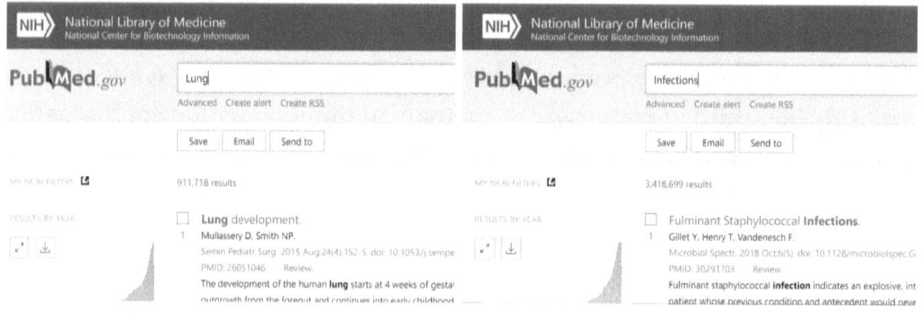

▲ **Figure 3.2:** Search results in PubMed when using separate queries for the keywords 'Lung' and 'Infections'

When a Boolean inquiry of 'Lung AND Infections' is used, the database returns 161,760 articles (see Figure 3.3) that contain both the keywords 'Lung' and 'Infections', removing all those articles that contain either 'Lung' or 'Infections' and returning only the articles that are specifically about infections of the lung.

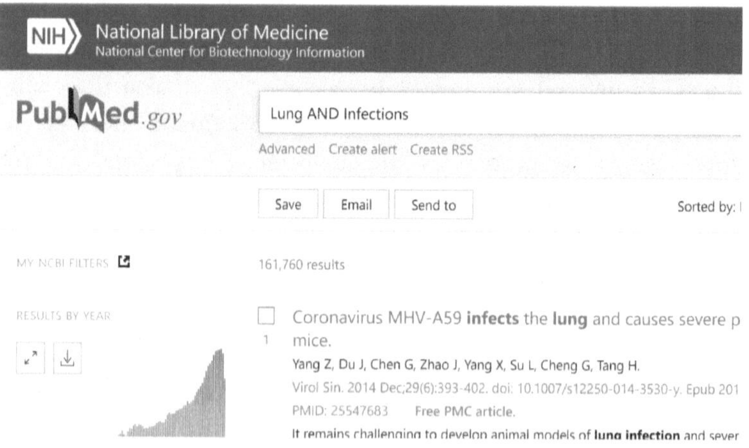

▲ **Figure 3.3:** Search results for the PubMed query: 'Lung AND Infections'

The query 'Lungs OR Infections' will return all items containing the words 'Lungs' or 'Infections'. Therefore, the search results will contain all the items about lungs and all the items about infections. So, the total number of results is 4,191,898 (Figure 3.4).

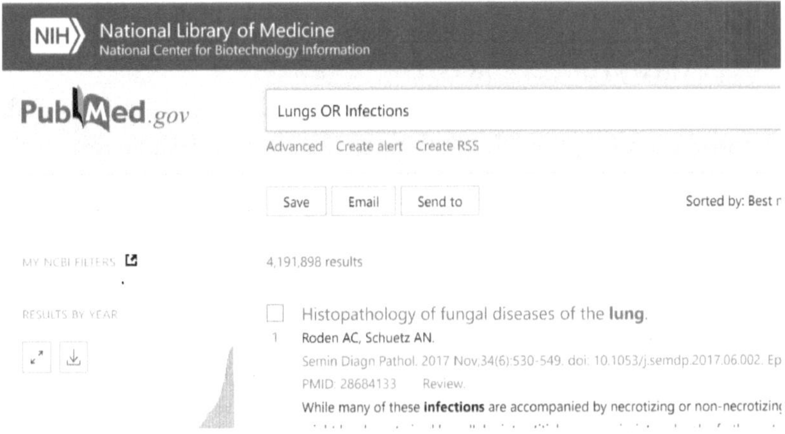

▲ **Figure 3.4:** Search results for the PubMed query: 'Lungs OR Infections'

Whereas, if the researcher gives the query 'Lungs NOT Infections', the search engine will retrieve only those items that are related to lungs, except infections. This search will remove all the infection-related items, returning only 773,199 articles (Figure 3.5).

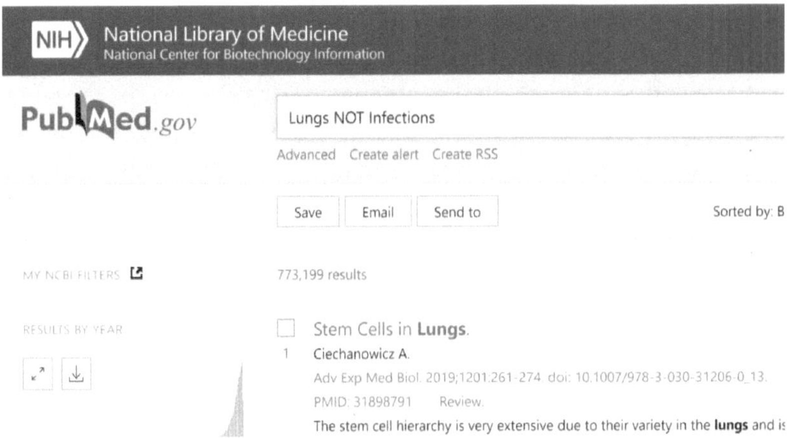

▲ **Figure 3.5:** Search results for the PubMed query: 'Lungs NOT Infections'

This basic demonstration is aimed to give researchers an idea of how Boolean queries work in a search engine like PubMed. However, this is not a structured or systematic way to search PubMed. Researchers may refer to the PubMed video tutorials to learn how to do MeSH searches.

3.7 SELECTING STUDIES FOR LITERATURE REVIEW

We have already discussed how to conduct a preliminary search in PubMed. The following points will highlight how to retrieve articles that are specifically related to the researcher's needs.

Step 1: Select articles specific to the need

Using a Boolean query or a structured query system, researchers have to collect specific articles related to their need. For example, if a researcher is using a Boolean query to search for lung and infection but wants only Randomized Controlled Trials (RCTs) of lung infections that have been published in the past five years, the researcher will have to apply the respective filters to retrieve the relevant articles. Once all the articles are retrieved, the researcher has to organise them, read them and review them.

Step 2: Select good-quality articles

Remember that the review of the retrieved articles should be scholarly and not too critical. For example, suppose a researcher is searching for literature about the therapeutic regimen for lung infections and finds out that articles are available only on researches that were conducted among the western population. This is a lacuna. In this manner, during the review, the researcher has to critically peruse through the existing evidence and find out the lacunae in the literature. Here, the researcher found that literature is available only for western population and not for Asian and Indian populations; the articles that reported about Indian populations were only quasi-experimental studies. This is the lacunae that the researcher has identified. Instead of finding faults in the literature, the researcher has identified new research areas.

Step 3: Review the methods of all retrieved articles

In this step, the researcher must compare the retrieved articles that they have chosen and summarise the different methods applied to a topic. This will give an idea about what methods the researchers have used in those studies. For example, if a researcher wants to conduct a study on a therapeutic regimen for lung infections, such review will help to identify specific methods that have been mentioned in those articles.

Step 4: Summarise the literature review in a tabular form

After reviewing all the selected articles, the researcher must summarise the key takeaways in a tabular form. This will help the researcher to organise the entire available literature and compare individual studies with one another.

Given below is an example of a literature review summary table (Table 3.1). The researcher can add or delete rows and columns in this table. The table may include details about citations, designs, objectives, study populations, sample size, measurable outcomes, study findings and conclusions. It is advisable to organise the table chronologically, meaning from recent to past. Thus, recent studies can be tabulated in the initial rows.

▼ **Table 3.1:** Summary of literature review

Citation with year	Study design	Objectives	Study population	Sample size	Measurable outcomes and results	Conclusions

3.8 WRITING A LITERATURE REVIEW

After organising the selected articles and tabulating them, the researcher can begin writing the literature review. There are three major parts to a literature review.

Introduction: In the introduction part of a literature review, the purpose and rationale of the review should be stated. This part should explain how the review was organised, how the queries were made and how the information was collected. It should explain the literature sequence, such as if it is from the most important to the least important, or from the earliest to the latest.

Empirical literature: The second part of the literature review should contain information about the included articles. It should speak about the quality of the studies that are relevant to the research question or topic. It should explain the strengths of each study in a paraphrased manner. Each of the studies should be appraised critically in a scholarly way so as to identify the lacunae or gaps in the study.

Summary: The researcher should summarise the entire literature review in this part. This part should recap the existing knowledge about the research question, the known and unknown information about the topic and the identified lacunae in the existing literature.

3.9 ETHICAL ISSUES IN LITERATURE REVIEW

Some ethical issues need to be taken care of while performing a literature review. Firstly, while extracting information from a manuscript or an article, the contents of the study should be presented honestly and without distortion. The studies should not be read in-between lines, and only the relevant part of the results should be taken.

Secondly, any weakness in the study should be stated in a scholarly manner; it should not be too critical. It should be addressed from a research point of view, from a scholarly point of view.

Finally, the sources of the selected literature should be accurately cited. Different referencing styles are available for documenting the citations of literature. Some of the most popular referencing styles are the Vancouver and Harvard styles.

Literature review should always be performed before initiating a study on a topic. The search results should be reviewed to identify new research areas. This chapter showed how to conduct a literature search in a database and provided an overview of how to write a literature review.

References and Further Reading

1. Corrall CJ, Wyer PC, Zick LS, Bockrath CR. How to find evidence when you need it, part 1: databases, search programs, and strategies. *Ann Emerg Med.* 2002;39(3):302-6.
2. Leite DFB, Padilha MAS, Cecatti JG. Approaching literature review for academic purposes: the literature review checklist. *Clinics.* 2019;74:e1403.
3. Ecker ED, Skelly AC. Conducting a winning literature search. *Evid Based Spine Care J.* 2010;1(1):9-14.

SECTION II

EPIDEMIOLOGICAL CONSIDERATIONS IN DESIGNING A RESEARCH STUDY

CHAPTER 04

MEASURES OF DISEASE FREQUENCY

R. Ramakrishnan

Learning Objectives

At the end of this chapter, readers will be able to:

1. List the commonly used measures of disease frequency
2. Define prevalence and incidence with respect to diseases
3. Describe the uses of prevalence and incidence measures
4. Recognise the relationship between incidence and prevalence

This chapter will discuss the indicators that are commonly used to measure disease frequency. Before moving on to discuss about the appropriate method of measuring disease frequency, let us first learn about 'population at risk'. **Population at risk** is the portion of the population that is susceptible to disease. It denotes the number of people who do not have a disease but are at a risk of developing it. Population at risk is described from the perspective of a disease or event, considering demographic and environmental factors. For example, the population at risk of developing cervical carcinoma is females in the age group of 30 to 70 years. As carcinoma of the cervix is mostly observed in women who are 30–70 years of age, the population at risk is females within this age group who do not have cervical cancer. Another example is hepatitis B virus (HBV) infection. The population at risk of developing hepatitis B are individuals in a geographic area who are HBV-negative but at risk of developing the infection. However, in some studies where everyone in the population is at risk of developing a particular disease, the total population is considered as the population at risk.

4.1 MEASURES OF DISEASE FREQUENCY

The common indicators of disease frequency are prevalence, incidence and case fatality. Prevalence and incidence are morbidity indicators, while case fatality is a mortality indicator.

4.2 PREVALENCE

Prevalence (P) is the **number of existing cases**, both old and new, in a defined population at a specific point in time. It is equal to the number of people with the disease in a specific geographic area at a specific point of time divided by the population at risk at the specific time and multiplied by a factor of 10.

$$\textit{Prevalence (P)} = \frac{\textit{Number of people with disease at a specific time}}{\textit{Population at risk at the specific time}} * 10^n$$

For example, a prevalence of 0.001 can be stated as 1 per 1000 or 10 per 10,000 or 100 per 100,000 if the value is multiplied by 1000, 10000 or 100000, depending on the size of the population at risk.

4.3 TYPES OF PREVALENCE

4.3.1 Point Prevalence

Point prevalence measures the **frequency of a disease at a given point in time**. It is like a snapshot. If P denotes prevalence, N denotes the population at the time 't', and C is the number of observed cases at time 't',

$$\textit{Point prevalence}(P) = \frac{C}{N}$$

For example, in a school, 150 children are screened for refractory errors at time t. The tests reveal that 15 children require glasses. The prevalence of refractory errors, in this case, is 15 divided by 150 or 0.1. Hence, the point prevalence of refractory error in this particular school is 10 per cent.

4.3.2 Period Prevalence

Period prevalence measures the **frequency of a disease over a period of time**. It is applicable when data has been collected over a period of time, and is denoted as PP. If C is the number of prevalent cases at the beginning of a time period, I is the number of incident cases that occur during the study period and N is the size of the population for the same time period, then period prevalence is equal to the sum of C and I divided by N.

$$\textbf{\textit{Period prevalence (PP)}} = \frac{C+I}{N}$$

For example, suppose you have a sample population of 150 persons, and you follow up on their medical condition for one year. At the beginning of your survey, 25 persons had the disease of interest and 15 new cases developed during the year. Here, we will calculate the point prevalence at the start of the period and period prevalence over time.

Point prevalence = 25/150 = 0.17 (17%)

Period prevalence = (25+15)/150 = 40/150 = 0.27 (27%)

4.4 FACTORS INFLUENCING PREVALENCE

Several factors influence the value of prevalence. The causes of increase and decrease in prevalence are presented in Table 4.1 below.

▼ **Table 4.1:** Causes of increase and decrease in prevalence

Causes of increase in prevalence	Causes of decrease in prevalence
Long duration of illness	Short duration of illness
Low cure rate	High cure rate
Low case fatality	High case fatality
Increase in new cases	Decrease in new cases
Immigration of patients	Emigration of patients
Improved detection	Improved cure rate
Emigration of healthy people	Immigration of healthy people

The prevalence of a disease can increase if there is an increase in the number of new cases. This may be due to immigration of patients, emigration of healthy people or a new, improved case detection mechanism. It could also increase because of long duration of the illness, low cure rate or low case fatality. For example, in the case of chronic diseases like diabetes mellitus, when insulin first became available, what happened to the prevalence of diabetes? The prevalence increased because diabetes was not cured but was controlled.

Many patients with diabetes who formerly would have died now survived; therefore, the prevalence increased.

The prevalence of a disease will decrease if the number of new cases decreases. This may be due to a high cure rate or high case fatality of the disease. In addition, if the duration of the illness decreases, prevalence tends to decrease. Decrease in prevalence could also occur if there is emigration of patients or immigration of healthy people. For example, if the prevalence of H1N1 influenza in a community is measured after an outbreak, it may be low or even zero, as all the H1N1 cases may be cured or might have died when the survey was conducted. Therefore, the prevalence may be close to zero.

Thus, changes in prevalence could be due to several reasons, which can be difficult to interpret. Researchers must study different aspects of population dynamics before interpreting the change in prevalence.

4.5 USES OF PREVALENCE

Prevalence data can be used to:

- **i.** Assess health care needs
- **ii.** Plan health services as it measures the burden of disease
- **iii.** Measure the occurrence of conditions with gradual onset
- **iv.** Study chronic diseases

4.6 INCIDENCE

Incidence is defined as the **number of new cases** recorded during a given period in a specific population.

Time is an important factor here. You must specify the time when you are presenting the incidence. Incidence measures the rapidity with which new cases occur in a population and can be expressed in absolute numbers in terms of **cumulative incidence** or **incidence density**.

4.7 TYPES OF INCIDENCE

4.7.1 Cumulative Incidence

Cumulative incidence is the number of new cases divided by the population at risk at the beginning of the study in a defined geographic area, multiplied by a factor of 10.

While calculating cumulative incidence, it is assumed that the entire population was at risk at the beginning and was followed up for a time period of observation.

$$\textbf{\textit{Cumulative incidence (CI)}} = \frac{\textit{Number of new cases}}{\textit{Population at risk at the beginning}} * 10^n$$

CI corresponds to the 'risk' of a health event. **Risk** is the probability that an individual will experience a health issue over a specified follow-up period, assuming that the individual neither had the disease initially nor died from other causes during follow-up.

4.7.2 Incidence Density

Incidence density, also known as **incidence rate**, is the number of new cases divided by the total person-time of observation, multiplied by a factor of 10.

$$\textbf{\textit{Incidence density (ID)}} = \frac{\textit{Total number of new cases}}{\textit{Total person} - \textit{time of observation}} * 10^n$$

The denominator of incidence rate or incidence density is person-time observed. **Person-time** is generally calculated based on a follow-up study wherein participants are followed up over time, and the occurrence of new incidences of the disease is reported. Person-time of observation is the **sum of the units of time each individual was at risk**. Typically, each participant is observed from an established starting time until one of four 'endpoints' is reached: onset of disease, death, migration out of the study (lost to follow-up) or end of the study.

Person-time is the sum of the time each person was observed, summed up for all persons. It is expressed as **person-years** or **person-months** or **person-days** or **person-hours of observation**. If one person at risk of disease is observed for one year, the person-time is '**1 person-year**'. Similarly, if one person at risk is observed for five years, then the person-time is 5 person-years. The person-time of five people at risk, each observed for only one year, is also 5 person-years. For example, in a study, five people were observed for five years. If all five participants were followed up for the entire five years of the study, then the denominator of incidence rate is equal to 25 person-years of observation.

4.8 USES OF INCIDENCE

Incidence data can be used to:

i. Describe the trends in disease or health events

ii. Evaluate the impact of prevention/control/intervention programs

4.9 CASE FATALITY

Case fatality relates the number of deaths due to a disease to the number of cases. To calculate case fatality, you need information on how many cases were there and how many of them died. Case fatality reflects the **severity of the disease**. It is the proportion of the number of deaths due to a disease or event to the total number of cases. Here, the numerator is the number of deaths due to a disease or event and the denominator is the total number of cases of the specific disease or event. It can be expressed as **proportion** or **ratio**.

$$\textbf{\textit{Case fatality ratio (CFR)}} = \frac{\textit{Number of deaths due to a disease / event among the incident cases}}{\textit{Total number of incident cases of the specific disease or event}}$$

4.10 RELATIONSHIP BETWEEN INCIDENCE AND PREVALENCE

The dynamics of incidence and prevalence is depicted in Figure 4.1. In a real-world situation, new cases continuously occur, and some cases cease to exist as a result of death or cure. The new cases that are pouring from the tap as shown in Figure 4.1 are incidence cases, whereas the cases remaining in the tank are the prevalence cases.

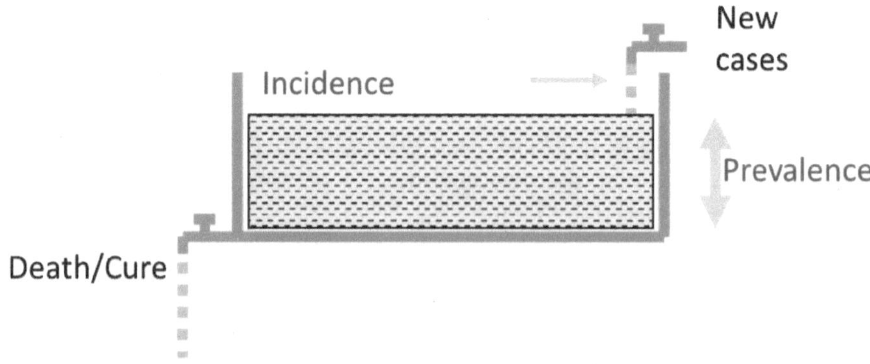

▲ **Figure 4.1:** Relationship between incidence and prevalence

Changes in prevalence from one time period to another can be caused by changes in the incidence rates, changes in the duration of disease or both. The relationship between 'Prevalence' and 'Incidence' is denoted using the following formula:

Prevalence (P) = Incidence (I) x Duration of the disease (D)

Duration of the disease can influence prevalence. A disease with a long duration of illness is likely to have a relatively large prevalence compared to a disease with a short duration of illness. For example, diabetes mellitus, which has a long latency period and no cure, has a high prevalence compared to common cold or influenza, which has a short duration of illness and is often cured. Therefore, diabetes is expected to have a high prevalence with a low incidence, while common cold or influenza will have a low prevalence with a high incidence.

References and Further Reading

1. Chapter 2 - Measuring health and disease. In: Bonita R, Beaglehole R, Kjellstrom T. Basic epidemiology. 2nd ed. Geneva: World Health Organization; 2006: p. 15-36. http://apps.who.int/iris/bitstream/10665/43541/1/9241547073_eng.pdf
2. Chapter 2 - Quantifying disease in populations. In: Coggon D, Rose G, Barker DJP. Epidemiology for the uninitiated. 4th ed. London: BMJ Publishing Group; 1997. http://www.bmj.com/about-bmj/resources-readers/publications/epidemiology-uninitiated/2-quantifying-disease-populations.
3. Chapter 3 - Descriptive epidemiological studies and clinical trials. In: World Health Organization. Health research methodology: a guide for training in research methods. Manila: WHO Regional Office for the Western Pacific; 2001: p.43-54.https://apps.who.int/iris/handle/10665/206929

CHAPTER 05

DESCRIPTIVE STUDY DESIGNS

Prabhdeep Kaur

Learning Objectives

At the end of this chapter, readers will be able to:

1. List the types of descriptive observational study designs
2. Describe the uses of descriptive study designs
3. Recognise the key elements of cross-sectional study designs

In this chapter, we are going to discuss descriptive study designs. Broadly, the epidemiological studies in health research can be divided into two categories: 'descriptive' and 'analytical' studies.

5.1 DESCRIPTIVE STUDY DESIGNS

A **descriptive study design** describes a disease state or an event in terms of person, place, time and the factors associated with the disease state or event. It focuses on what (health issue) is happening among whom (person), where (place) and when (time). It also describes how (modes of transmission) and why (risk factors) a disease is occurring in a specific population.

Types of Descriptive Studies

Descriptive studies can be of two types. One is the studies conducted on individuals, and the other is the studies conducted on populations. Studies that are conducted on populations are called '**ecological studies**'. At the individual level, various types of studies can be conducted, such as case reports, case series and cross-sectional surveys.

We will cover four main types of descriptive studies in this chapter—case reports, case series, ecological studies and cross-sectional surveys. Figure 5.1 below shows the classification of epidemiological study designs. You will learn about all of these study designs in the coming pages.

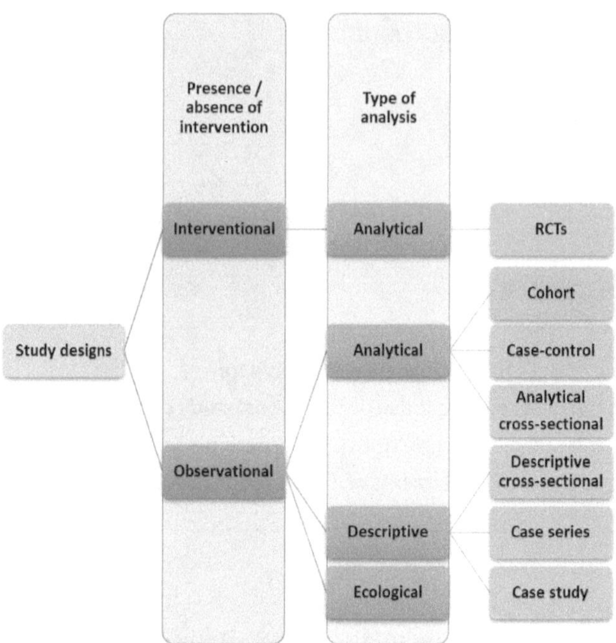

▲ **Figure 5.1:** Classification of epidemiological study designs

5.1.1 Case Reports

A '**case report**' is a detailed description of a single case. It means reporting a particular clinical manifestation or an interesting phenomenon that you found in your clinic or laboratory. Case reports are extremely useful for sharing your experience about new diseases, familiar diseases and rare manifestations. Case reports can be used to generate hypotheses about pathophysiological mechanisms or document clinical findings.

Case reports are usually published in peer-reviewed journals under a separate section with details about the clinical condition, the type of case report, existing evidence and available literature.

5.1.2 Case Series

In **case series**, we study a relatively larger group of patients who have a particular disease. This type of study is based on a series of specific cases and does not use any comparison group. Case series can help researchers understand or develop a clinical picture of patients presenting with a specific disease.

Example 1: In a case series, we may study 10 or more patients who have a rare type of cancer. This can help us understand whether the kinds of findings that we observe are really due to the disease or due to chance. The only problem with this case series is that you do not have a comparison group.

Example 2: In 1981, a case series was conducted on pneumocystis pneumonia, which was observed in five homosexual men. This helped researchers understand how pneumocystis pneumonia, which is not a very common condition, was occurring in the same kind of individuals. This study subsequently led to the discovery of AIDS.

5.1.3 Ecological Studies

Ecological study is a type of study in which the unit of study or analysis is a 'group'. In this type of studies, we do not collect information on the distribution of exposure and disease at the individual level; rather, we do it at the country level, population level or regional level. We collect information at the population level and try to understand a health event by relating the population to the problem. Thus, we would not have individual-level data but can study groups of population.

Example: Consider the research question, "What is the average intake of fat among people living in Tamil Nadu?" This study can help us learn about the incidence of cardiovascular disease in the population. However, we would only know the fat intake at the population level, not at the individual level. This information will help us generate a hypothesis and then correlate it with the incidence of cardiovascular disease. Another example is collecting information about the per capita consumption of fat in every state and then correlating it with the incidence of cardiovascular disease. Then, we can determine whether the states with higher per capita consumption of fat also have higher rates of coronary artery disease. If we find a correlation, we could conduct another detailed study to understand whether there is a correlation between fat intake and cardiovascular disease at the individual level.

5.1.4 Cross-Sectional Surveys

This is the most common type of study. We are all aware of the '**Census**'. A census is a cross-sectional survey that is conducted every 10 years, across the whole country. **Cross-sectional survey** is an observation of a cross-section of a population at a single point of time.

A cross-sectional survey captures a set of information about a population or an individual at a particular point of time. Cross-sectional studies are extremely useful for gauging the magnitude or burden of a problem. For example, if we want to know the burden of high blood pressure in a community, for which we collect information at a particular point of time, it is called a cross-sectional survey. Census is an example of a cross-sectional study that covers the entire population of the country. During the census, data collectors visit every house and enquire about the number of members in the family, their education, occupation and so on. But this information is collected for a particular year, say 2011. So, it may not be true for 2012.

However, all surveys are not done like the census. In most surveys, a sample of the population is selected, as it is not possible to survey one billion people for everything. For example, for the National Family Health Survey, a sample of the study population is selected, and data are collected from that sample alone. Surveying the sample population at a given point of time will help the researchers understand the magnitude of a problem in the study population.

Similarly, it is not possible for a clinician to include all patients in a study. In this situation, the researcher needs to select a sample. In subsequent chapters, the sample size and sampling method for cross-sectional surveys will be discussed. The researcher can also collect data on various types of 'exposure' or 'outcome' from the sample. '**Exposure**' refers to the different types of risk factors, while '**outcome**' refers to the disease or the event of interest. For example, in a study conducted to determine the burden of high blood pressure and the risk factors associated with it, high blood pressure is the 'outcome' and behavioural risk factors such as obesity, smoking and drinking are 'exposures'. Therefore, the survey will include questions on the participants' history of blood pressure, smoking, alcohol consumption and anthropometric measurements like height, weight and other potential exposures.

Uses of Cross-Sectional Surveys

- Cross-sectional surveys measure the 'burden of disease' or 'prevalence of disease'. For example, we can survey a random group of 100 people in a community and find out how many of them have high blood pressure. Alternatively, we can measure their blood pressure using a sphygmomanometer/digital blood pressure machine and identify those who have a high blood pressure. Based on this value, we can calculate the prevalence of high blood pressure in the community.

- It can also be used to measure the burden of risk factors. For example, we can survey the same 100 people and ask them about behavioural risk factors like smoking and alcohol intake. This information will help in identifying the burden of risk factors.
- It helps in understanding the distribution of a health problem by time, place and person. For example, if we are enquiring about diarrhoea in a village, who has suffered, in which part of the village it is occurring and in which period of the year it is occurring, it will give us an idea about the distribution of the health problem (diarrhoea).
- It can provide useful information for planning health services. Suppose, on enquiring about diarrhoea, we find that it is more common among children under the age of five. This information will help the health service provider to modify the plan of health service delivery in the village so that diarrhoea in children can be prevented or managed.
- At the state, country or global level, cross-sectional surveys help us set priorities for disease control. For example, at the central level, policymakers may have the question: In which disease should they invest their resources? To prioritise their resources, they have to know the magnitude of the health problems in the country. A cross-sectional survey will help researchers identify the magnitude of a particular health problem. However, cross-sectional surveys are not ideal for testing hypotheses. Hypotheses testing can be done using analytical studies. A cross-sectional study mainly helps us to generate hypotheses.
- Cross-sectional studies sometimes help to understand the effectiveness of an intervention. For example, suppose a new drug is introduced into the usual regimen of a disease. In this case, we can measure the patient outcome both before and after implementing the intervention by conducting a cross-sectional study.

5.1.5 Analytical or Comparative Cross-Sectional Study

When a cross-sectional study examines at least two groups and focuses on comparing the groups and describing them, it is known as an **analytical cross-sectional study**.

For example, a study on hypertension may be conducted to achieve the following objectives:

- To estimate the proportion of hypertension in a community
- To establish potential behavioural (smoking, alcohol, unhealthy diet) or biological (overweight/obesity) risk factors of hypertension in the community

In this case, the researcher not only describes the variables under study but also compares hypertensive and non-hypertensive people and tries to understand which of these risk factors might have contributed more to hypertension. This type of cross-sectional study is called an analytical cross-sectional study.

Advantages of Cross-Sectional Studies

- Cross-sectional studies are relatively easy to perform compared to other study designs.
- Cross-sectional studies can be planned and completed within a short period of time.
- Cross-sectional studies are less expensive.

Limitations of Cross-Sectional Studies

- Cross-sectional studies are not useful for studying disease aetiology.
- Hypotheses cannot be tested using cross-sectional studies.
- Cross-sectional studies are not suitable for the study of rare diseases.

Another major limitation of a cross-sectional study is that we cannot comment on what happened first—the exposure or the outcome. For example, while conducting a survey on hypertension, we measure all prevalent hypertensive cases irrespective of the starting point of the disease. Moreover, when we ask people about their smoking habit or alcohol intake, the response may be only 'Yes' or 'No'. Here also, we are not considering the time of origin of the habits. We do not know whether hypertension happened first or smoking happened first. Similarly, if you study obesity and diabetes in a cross-sectional survey, you may find people who are diabetic as well as obese. However, you would not know what happened first, diabetes or obesity.

5.2 EXAMPLES OF RESEARCH QUESTIONS THAT CAN BE ADDRESSED THROUGH CROSS-SECTIONAL SURVEYS

Let us now see some examples of research questions that can be answered through a cross-sectional study. A researcher can use a cross-sectional study to estimate the prevalence of hypertension in a city. A clinician in a primary health centre (PHC) can conduct a cross-sectional study to understand patient satisfaction or the utilisation pattern of medical services in the health facility. This type of study is called '**exit survey**'. Cross-sectional studies can be done in any setting—they could be done in schools, health facilities, the community or at the clinical level.

However, while interpreting the findings of the study, the researcher needs to be cautious. The researcher should keep in mind that the 'exposure' and 'outcome' cannot be linked in a cross-sectional study, as they are measured simultaneously.

Case reports and case series are extremely useful to clinicians for documenting uncommon clinical manifestations in a certain set of patients. Ecological studies will be useful when group-level data is required to relate and generate a hypothesis. A cross-sectional study is the most common study design that is used for measuring the burden or magnitude of health conditions.

References and Further Reading

1. CDC. Pneumocystis Pneumonia - Los Angeles. Morbidity and Mortality Weekly Report (MMWR). 1981; 30(21): 2.
2. Levin KA. Study Design VI - Ecological studies. *Evid Based Dent.* 2006;7(4):108.
3. Stokes V, Fertleman C. Writing a case report in 10 steps. *BMJ.*2015; 350:2693.
4. Murad MH, Sultan S, Haffar S, Bazerbachi F. Methodological quality and synthesis of case series and case reports. *BMJ Evid Based Med.* 2018;23(2):60–3.
5. Setia MS. Methodology Series Module 3: Cross-sectional studies. *Indian J Dermatol.* 2016;61(3):261–4.

CHAPTER 06

ANALYTICAL STUDY DESIGNS

Manoj V. Murhekar

Learning Objectives

At the end of this chapter, readers will be able to:

1. List the types of analytical observational study designs
2. Recognise the key elements of a cohort study design
3. Describe the key elements of a case-control study design

In the previous chapter, you learned that epidemiological studies can be categorised as **descriptive** and **analytical study designs**. Epidemiological studies can also be divided into two categories based on the exposure assigned to the study—experimental study and observational study. In **experimental studies**, the researcher assigns the exposure. The exposure could be a new intervention, a new drug or a new vaccine. Experimental studies are further classified as '**randomised**' and '**non-randomised studies**', based on the randomised allocation of exposure. On the other hand, in **observational studies**, the researcher does not assign any exposure. Observational studies that do not have any comparison group are called '**descriptive studies**'. In these studies, health events in terms of person, place and time are described. If there is a comparison group in the observational studies, they are called '**analytical studies**'. In this chapter, two types of analytical studies —cohort and case-control studies will be discussed.

A **cohort study** progresses from exposure to outcome, while a **case-control study** progresses from outcome to exposure. Therefore, in analytical studies, the researcher carefully measures the pattern of exposure and disease in the population, and, using comparison, makes inferences about the exposure and disease.

6.1 COHORT STUDY

The word 'cohort' has a military origin, rather than a medical origin. In the Roman army, a 300–600-man unit was called a cohort, whereas, in epidemiology, the word '**cohort**' refers to a group of individuals who share some common characteristics. For example, all the children born today will form today's birth cohort.

6.1.1 Design of Cohort Studies

Cohort studies progress **from exposure to outcome**. For example, look at Figure 6.1. A researcher wants to study the relationship between cigarette smoking and the development of cardiovascular disease. Here, the exposure is cigarette smoking and the outcome is the development of cardiovascular disease.

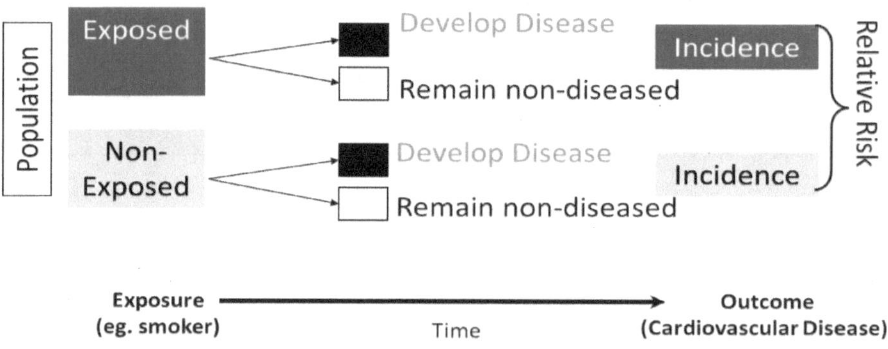

Figure 6.1: Framework of a cohort study

Cohort studies begin with the selection of exposed and unexposed cohorts. In this example, it would be smokers and non-smokers. After selection, these cohorts will be followed up for a predetermined period of time. Some of the exposed and unexposed participants may develop cardiovascular disease, while the remaining cohorts remain non-diseased. After making these inferences, the researcher will calculate the incidence of cardiovascular disease in the exposed population and the unexposed population, and then compare this incidence by using a measure of association called '**Relative Risk**'.

6.1.2 Types of Cohort Studies

There are three types of cohort studies:

1. Prospective cohort study
2. Retrospective cohort study
3. Ambispective cohort study

Prospective Cohort Study

In a prospective cohort study, the exposure and disease would not have occurred at the start of the study.

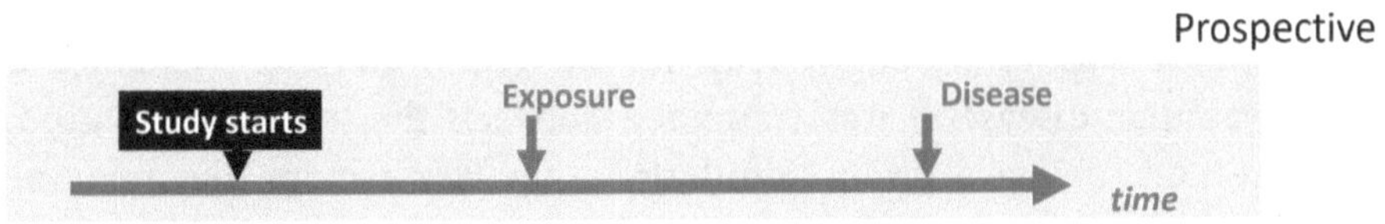

Prospective

Study starts
Exposure
Disease
time

▲ **Figure 6.2:** Prospective cohort study

Retrospective Cohort Study

In a retrospective cohort study, both exposure and disease would have already occurred before the start of the study.

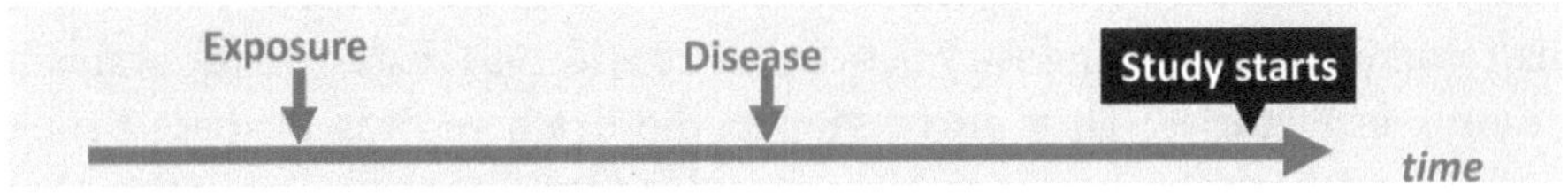

▲ **Figure 6.3:** Retrospective cohort study

Ambispective Cohort Study

When there is a combination of both prospective and retrospective cohort designs, it is called

a bi-directional study or an ambispective cohort study. In this study design, when the study starts, the exposure would have already occurred, and the researcher will follow the exposed and unexposed individuals until they develop the outcome.

Ambispective

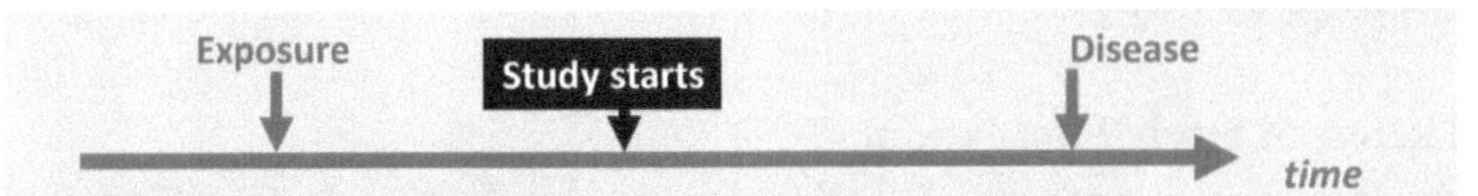

▲ **Figure 6.4:** Ambispective cohort study

6.1.3 Examples of Different Types of Cohort Studies

Framingham Heart Study

The Framingham heart study is one of the oldest prospective cohort studies that was initiated in 1948. The objective of this study was to identify risk factors for cardiovascular disease. This study was conducted in the town of Framingham, which had a population of about 28,000 people. A sample of this population was divided into two groups, based on those who had risk factors and those who did not. The researchers considered several risk factors, one of them being hypertension. They classified the population into those who had hypertension and those who did not have hypertension. This cohort was then followed up for 20 years, and the incidence of cardiovascular disease(s) was compared between the hypertensive group and the normotensive group. Similarly, other risk factors like smoking, obesity, inadequate physical activity, increased blood pressure and elevated cholesterol were compared.

Aniline Dyes and Urinary Bladder Cancer

This is an example of a retrospective cohort study. The objective of this study was to evaluate the role of aniline dyes in the development of urinary bladder cancer. For this study, the researchers examined 4,622 deceased people who had worked in the dye industry between 1920 and 1951, based on the available records in factories. They also reviewed the death records of these people and checked for the presence of urinary bladder tumours. Thereafter, they compared the rates of bladder cancer-related deaths in this population with that of the expected number of bladder cancer-related deaths using national statistics. In this case, the 'exposure' and 'outcome' had already occurred before the initiation of the study.

6.1.4 Stages of a Cohort Study

A cohort study is conducted in four stages:

a) Selection of study population
b) Gathering of baseline information
c) Follow-up of cohort
d) Analysis of outcome

a) **Selection of Study Population**

There are two approaches to selecting the study population. The first approach is selecting a cohort from the general population, as was done in the *Framingham cohort study*, or selecting a subset of the general population, as was done in the *Nurses' health study*. The second approach is selecting a special exposure group, such as occupational groups.

Comparison groups in a cohort study can be either internal or external.

- **Internal Comparison Group**
  In a cohort study, the unexposed people in the study population could be considered as an internal comparison group. For example, in the Framingham cohort study, the study participants who had hypertension were considered as exposed population, whereas those who had normal blood pressure were considered as the unexposed population.
- **External Comparison Group**
  Sometimes, it is not possible to have an internal comparison group within the study design. For example, in the aniline dye and urinary bladder cancer study, every workman who had worked in the dye industry was exposed, and so it was not possible to have an internal comparison group. Therefore, the researchers compared the death rates of bladder cancer due to aniline exposure with that of the general population. In such situations, they could use an external comparison group.

b) **Gathering of Baseline Information**
Once you select the study population, the next step is to collect baseline information about the study population. The objective of this step is to assess the exposure status of the cohort participants. Based on the baseline information of the study population, the researcher could exclude those individuals who have the disease of interest at the baseline level, so that the population that remains would be the ones who are at risk of developing the disease. At the same time, the researcher can also collect data about other exposure variables.

c) **Follow–Up of Cohort**
Once the recruitment of the exposed and unexposed population has been completed, the next step is to follow up on the study population. There are three principles for doing a good follow-up. First, having uniform surveillance in exposed and unexposed groups; second, completing the ascertainment of exposure and outcomes; and third, using standardised methods for the diagnosis of outcomes.

d) **Analysis of Outcome**
The 2×2 table used in a cohort study would look like the one below (Table 6.1).

▼ **Table 6.1:** Presentation of data in a 2×2 table in a cohort study

	Diseased	Non-diseased	Total
Exposed	a	b	a+b
Unexposed	c	d	c+d
	a+c	b+d	a+b+c+d

Known at the start of the study

Let us look at an example to understand the table better. A researcher started a study by selecting people who were exposed to the disease, which is a+b, and the people who were unexposed, which is c+d. She/he then followed up with these people. a+c developed the disease, while b+d remained non-diseased. Therefore, at the beginning of the study, the researcher knew who was exposed and who was not exposed (Table 6.1).

6.1.5 Relative Risk (RR)

As a cohort study includes both exposed and unexposed groups, the risk of developing the disease among these groups can be calculated separately. The ratio of these two risks is known as the **Relative Risk (RR)** of a disease.

Incidence of disease in exposed population = a/a+b

Incidence of disease in unexposed population = c/c+d

The ratio of these two incidences is relative risk.

$$\textbf{\textit{Relative Risk (RR)}} = \frac{\textit{Incidence of disease among exposed population}\left(\dfrac{a}{a+b}\right)}{\textit{Incidence of disease among unexposed population}\left(\dfrac{c}{c+d}\right)}$$

Interpreting Relative Risk

If the relative risk is one (**RR=1**), it means that the incidence of disease in the exposed and unexposed population is the same, and the researcher can interpret this as, the exposure not being associated with the disease. If the relative risk is more than one (**RR>1**), the incidence of the disease is higher in the exposed population as compared to the unexposed population. Hence, the exposure is positively associated with the disease. If the relative risk is less than one (**RR<1**), it means that the incidence of disease in the exposed population is lower than in the unexposed population. Therefore, exposure is negatively associated with the disease.

6.1.6 Strengths and Weaknesses of a Cohort Study

Strengths

i. Cohort studies allow the calculation of incidence. At the start of the study, the researcher selects the exposed population and unexposed population. After following them up for a certain period, the researcher can calculate the incidence of the disease.

ii. In cohort studies, multiple outcomes can be examined for a given exposure.

iii. In cohort studies, the temporality of the disease can be assessed.

iv. Cohort studies are useful in cases of rare exposure.

Weaknesses

i. Cohort studies could be expensive and time-consuming. The sample size of these studies could be large, and participants need to be followed up for a long period of time.

ii. Cohort studies are not recommended for rare diseases or diseases that have a long latency period.

iii. If the study participants are not followed up carefully in both the groups, then a differential loss to follow up could happen, which could bias the study results.

6.2 CASE-CONTROL STUDY

Case-control studies are the exact opposite of cohort studies with respect to the direction or logic of the study.

6.2.1 Design of Case-Control Study

Let us learn about the design of a case-control study by looking at an example of a case-control study conducted by Doll and Hill. The objective of this study was to test the association between cigarette smoking and lung cancer. For their study, Doll and Hill selected lung cancer patients who were admitted in about 20 hospitals in London. All these patients had histopathologically proven cases of lung cancer. For each case of lung cancer, they selected a control, which was a non-lung cancer patient admitted in the same hospital. These cases and controls were then interviewed to find out their prior exposures. By using a detailed questionnaire, Doll and Hill found out how many people had a history of cigarette smoking, how many of them were currently smoking, at what age they started smoking and the type of cigarette smoking.

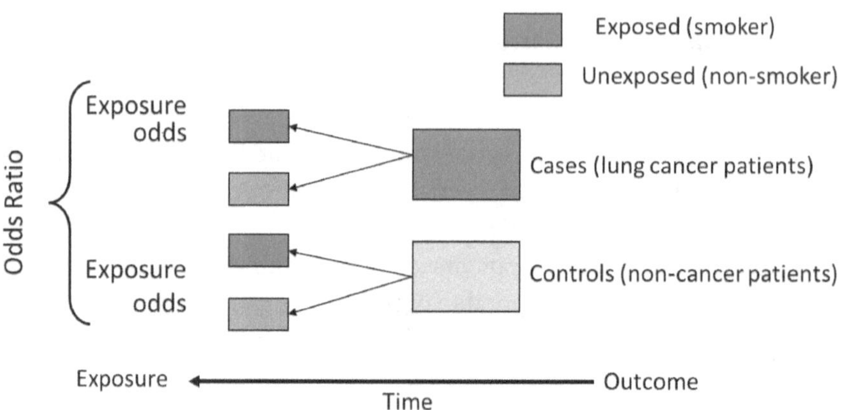

▲ **Figure 6.5:** Framework of a case-control study

The first step was selecting the cases. In this study, Doll and Hill found out how many of the cases and controls were exposed to cigarette smoking and how many were unexposed. Based on this data, they calculated the 'exposure odds among cases' and 'exposure odds among controls'. Then, they calculated the 'Odds Ratio' as a measure of association between exposure and outcome (Figure 6.5).

6.2.2 Stages of a Case-Control Study

There are four important stages in a case-control study:

a) Selection of cases
b) Selection of controls
c) Collection of valid information about exposures
d) Analysis

a) Selection of Cases

Theoretically, all people in the source population who develop the disease of interest could be included in the study. However, most researchers use samples from the population. One point that should be kept in mind is that the selection of cases should be independent of exposure to the disease. The researcher must have a clear definition of the outcome to be studied and should also decide whether to include prevalent or incident cases. Prevalent cases are those cases that already occurred in the past, whereas incident cases are the newly occurring ones.

So, if you take the prevalent cases, they will be readily available; by including them, you can save time and money. Despite these advantages, it is generally recommended to include incident cases mainly because prevalent cases may be related more to the survival of the disease than the development of the disease.

Sources of Cases

There are two important sources for the selection of cases. One is a hospital or clinic. It is easier to find cases in hospitals and clinics. However, cases admitted in hospitals may be more severe and may not represent the cases in the community.

The other source is population. For example, in the cancer registry, you would find cases that are more likely to represent the source population because they are not biased by factors that draw patients to a particular hospital.

b) **Selection of Controls**

The second stage of the case-control study is the selection of controls. Controls are the people who do not have the disease under investigation. Controls represent the distribution of exposure in the source population. They provide insight about the background rate of exposure in the population from which the cases are selected. Controls should also be selected independent of the exposure status.

Sources of Controls

There are three sources of control. The first source is the population, wherein samples will be selected from the general population. The second source is healthcare facilities. In the study conducted by Doll and Hill, the controls were selected from a healthcare facility. The third source is cases collected from friends circle or neighbourhoods.

c) **Collection of Valid Information About Exposures**

Once the cases and controls are selected, the next important task is collecting relevant data about past exposures. There are three important principles for collecting data on exposures. The data should be collected i) objectively, so that the measurements are reproducible; ii) accurately, so that the information reflects the actual effect of exposure as closely as possible and iii) precisely, to ensure quality management in exposure measurement.

d) **Analysis**

The 2×2 table in a case-control study will be as presented below (Table 6.2).

▼ **Table 6.2:** Presentation of data in a 2×2 table in a case-control study

	Cases	Controls	Total
Exposed	a	b	a+b
Unexposed	c	d	c+d
	a+c	b+d	a+b+c+d

Known at the start of the study

In case-control studies, the cases and controls will be known at the start of the study. In the given example, a+c were the cases to start with and b+d were the controls. Among the cases (a+c), 'a' were exposed and 'c' were unexposed, and among the controls (b+d), 'b' were exposed and 'd' were unexposed (Table 6.2).

6.2.3 **Odds Ratio (OR)**

In a case-control study, the incidence of disease cannot be calculated. But another measure of the association between the disease and its incidence, known as the **Odds Ratio (OR)**, can be calculated. The odds of an event is the ratio of the probability of having a disease to the probability of not having the disease. Hence, the odds of a case being exposed is the probability that the case was exposed divided by the probability that the case was not exposed (Table 6.3).

▼ **Table 6.3:** Odds Ratio estimation using a 2×2 table in a case-control study

	Cases	Controls	Total
Exposed	a	b	a+b
Unexposed	c	d	c+d
	a+c	b+d	a+b+c+d

$$\textit{Odds that a case was exposed} = \frac{\textit{Probability that the case was exposed}}{\textit{Probability that the case was not exposed}}$$

= (a/a+c)/(c/a+c)

= a/c

$$\textbf{\textit{Odds that a control was exposed}} = \frac{\textit{Probability that the control was exposed}}{\textit{Probability that the control was not exposed}}$$

= (b/b+d)/(d/b+d)
= b/d

The ratio of these two odds is known as the odds ratio.
So, odds ratio = (a/c)/(b/d) = ad/bc.

Interpreting the Odds Ratio
Similar to relative risk, odds ratio can be interpreted in three ways.

If the odds ratio is one (**OR=1**), it indicates that the odds of exposure among cases and controls are the same; so, the researcher can conclude that exposure is not associated with the disease. If the odds ratio is more than one (**OR>1**), it indicates that the odds of exposure among cases are higher than that among controls; so, the researcher can conclude that exposure is positively associated with the disease. If the odds ratio is less than one (**OR<1**), the odds of exposure among cases are lower than that among controls; so, the researcher can conclude that exposure is negatively associated with the disease.

6.2.4 Strengths and Weaknesses of Case-Control Studies

Strengths

- **i.** Case-control studies are useful in the case of rare diseases or when the disease has a long latency period.
- **ii.** These studies are easy, quick to conduct and inexpensive.
- **iii.** They require relatively fewer participants than cohort studies.
- **iv.** In a case-control study, multiple exposures or risk factors can be examined simultaneously.

Weaknesses

- **i.** Case-control studies are susceptible to several biases; recall bias is one of the most important biases.
- **ii.** Selecting an appropriate comparison group can sometimes be difficult in a case-control study.
- **iii.** Incidence of disease cannot be determined in a case-control study.

References and Further Reading

1. Chapter 2 - Research strategies and design. In: World Health Organization. Health research methodology: a guide for training in research methods. Manila: WHO Regional Office for the Western Pacific; 2001: p.11-42.
2. Mann CJ. Observational research methods. Research design II: cohort, cross-sectional, and case-control studies. Emerg MedJ2003; 20:54-60.
3. Levin KA. Study design V. Case-control studies. Evid Based Dent 2006;7(3):834.
4. Levin KA. Study design IV. Cohort studies. Evid Based Dent 2006;7(2):51-2.

EXPERIMENTAL STUDY DESIGNS: CLINICAL TRIALS

Sanjay Mehendale

Learning Objectives

At the end of this chapter, readers will be able to:

1. Describe the basic concepts related to randomised controlled trials
2. Define the purpose of randomisation, blinding and ethical issues related to experimental study design
3. Identity and classify different types of trial designs

7.1 OVERVIEW OF STUDY DESIGNS

As explained earlier, epidemiological study designs are classified as observational and experimental study designs (Figure 7.1).

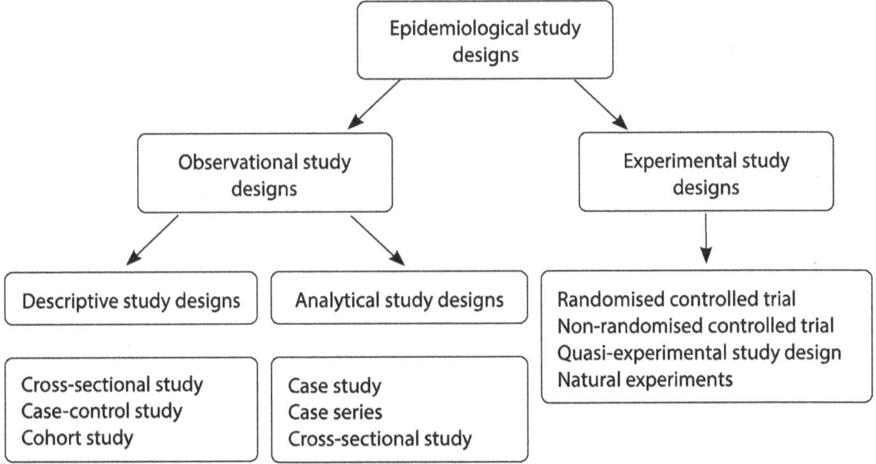

▲ **Figure 7.1:** Classification of epidemiological study designs

An observational study is a type of study design in which the researcher observes the chain of events without actively intervening; in other words, the 'exposure' is not assigned by the researcher. Depending on the nature of the study, observational study designs can be broadly classified as descriptive and analytical study designs.

Descriptive studies include case-series, cross-sectional descriptive studies, and ecological studies. Analytical studies include cross-sectional analytical studies, case-control studies that are usually retrospective and cohort studies that are prospective. Both these have been described in chapters 5 and 6.

An experimental study design is one in which the exposure is assigned by the researcher. Clinical trials are a classic example of experimental study design. Clinical trials are regarded as one of the main scientific advances in clinical research methods in the last century. They are considered the methodological standard of excellence and described as the gold standard for scientific experiments.

7.2 SIGNIFICANCE OF CLINICAL TRIALS

Clinical trials are essential for generating evidence to translate the results of basic scientific research into ways to prevent, diagnose or treat a particular disease or condition. They have a huge translational value. Trials involving human participants are designed to answer scientific questions and find better ways to prevent, diagnose or treat a disease.

7.3 RANDOMISED CONTROLLED CLINICAL TRIALS

A randomised controlled clinical trial is a **planned experiment** that is primarily designed to assess the efficacy of prophylactic, diagnostic or therapeutic agents. It also helps in testing the efficacy of new devices, different drug regimens or new procedures such as investigative procedures in human participants.

It essentially involves **comparing the outcomes** of a trial in two groups of individuals suffering from a particular disease of interest. For example, in therapeutic trials, we compare the outcomes among patients with comparable characteristics by varying the intervention. One group receives a new treatment, while the other group receives the standard treatment. Both these groups are then followed up and evaluated over a period of time. This is a **prospective study** in which patients in both the groups, one treated or exposed to intervention and the other given the standard treatment are followed over the same period to find out how many of them get effectively cured.

In a randomised controlled clinical trial, the researcher manipulates or modifies the environment, and then follows the participants in both the groups for a pre-determined period of time. The researcher uses various techniques to decide whether the participants should be placed in the control arm receiving the standard drug or the intervention arm receiving a new drug. Randomisation is a technique that is used to assign individuals to groups in trials. This concept will be discussed later on in this book.

7.4 OBJECTIVES OF CLINICAL TRIALS

Clinical trials can be employed in a variety of scenarios. Clinical trials are normally conducted to evaluate new forms of therapy or prevention methods, such as:

- New drugs or treatments
- New medical or healthcare technologies
- New organisation or delivery systems of health care
- New methods of primary prevention
- New programmes for screening or early detection of diseases

7.5 SCHEMATICS OF A THERAPEUTIC CLINICAL TRIAL

7.5.1 Therapeutic Scenario

Usually, clinical trials are used to test drugs and pharmaceuticals that have therapeutic benefits.

A novice researcher may wonder, "How are these trials conducted?"

Here is an example of how clinical trials are conducted. Suppose there are a large number of individuals suffering from a particular disease. A researcher wants to determine whether a new treatment regimen for the disease could help achieve a better cure rate. The researcher will take a sample of the individuals suffering from the disease who are eligible to participate in a clinical trial. This sample may not be representative of the total population. The researcher must then confirm that these eligible patients are willing to participate in the trial. The eligible and willing participants will then be assigned to two different arms through randomisation technique, which will be discussed later in this chapter. The patients in one arm will receive the new or first type of treatment, while the patients in the other arm will receive the standard or second type of treatment. Then, the patients in both the groups will be followed up for a pre-defined duration. The frequency of the follow-up may be once every three months, once every six months, once a year or once in two years, depending on the research scenario. The patients in both the groups will then be assessed to determine the number of patients cured of the disease and those who continue to have the disease.

Clinical trials are useful in quantifying and analysing the anticipated benefit of a new treatment in terms of the cure rate for a particular disease, compared to the standard or old treatment.

7.5.2 Prevention Scenario

Clinical trials can be used in **prevention scenarios**, such as for testing the efficacy of a new vaccine. Here, the eligible population comprises individuals susceptible to or at risk of developing a particular disease. Like in a therapeutic trial, the researcher will take a sample of eligible individuals who are willing to participate in the trial and divide them into two arms in a randomised manner: One arm will receive the new vaccine, while the other will receive a placebo or some other type of vaccine. It is important to discuss at length whether a placebo or some other type of vaccine will be given to the control arm or the comparator arm. These two groups of individuals will then be followed up for a certain period of time at pre-defined intervals, to determine how many of them in both the arms actually acquire the disease in question.

If the vaccine is effective, fewer people will acquire the disease in the new vaccine arm than in the control, comparator or placebo arm. The researcher can analyse this difference in efficacy statistically and decide whether the new vaccine would be effective in preventing the occurrence of that particular disease in susceptible populations.

7.6 RANDOMISATION

Randomisation is the most critical step in a clinical trial. It is a process in which all eligible participants have an equal chance of being assigned to any study arm or group. There may be two or more arms in any trial. The number of participants in each arm is decided *a priori*. The participants are then assigned to various arms in a predetermined manner. It is important to note that the participants cannot choose the arm to which they would be assigned. The assignment is done through a neutral process. Besides, the investigators also do not decide whether a particular participant goes in arm A or arm B, or the intervention arm or the control arm. Through randomisation, the participants are assigned to one group or another.

One group receives the widely accepted treatment, called the standard treatment or the gold standard, while the other group receives the new treatment that is being tested. The researchers run the trial with the hope that the newer treatment will be better than the standard treatment.

Randomisation is the best way to validate the effectiveness of a new agent or intervention by ensuring that all groups are as similar as possible. It also minimises confounding, co-interventions and bias in outcome ascertainment.

7.7 BLINDING

Two problems generally arise in trials—**co-intervention** and **biased outcome ascertainment**. Let us first learn about co-intervention using an example. If the participants of a trial are aware of the allocation groups, they may want to exchange groups; if it is a behavioural response, they may modify their behaviour despite being in the control arm. In some instances, this may be facilitated by a staff involved in the study, medical providers, family or friends etc. Such co-intervention can vitiate the results of the trial.

Now, let us learn about biased outcome ascertainment using an example. If a patient knows that they are receiving a new drug, they may exaggerate any minor adverse effects that they may be facing. On the other hand, if the patient receives the standard treatment, they may not report any side effects. Similarly, personnel involved in ascertaining the outcomes of study participants may or may not report the adverse effects if they know the allocation groups.

Both these pitfalls can be minimised by blinding. **Blinding** is a quality improvement technique that is often used in clinical trials. It is a procedure in which the allocation of participants to intervention or control groups is kept concealed. Blinding can be of three types, depending on whether the participant, investigator and/or the statistician is kept unaware of the allocated groups. When participants are unaware of their allocated treatment group, i.e., they do not know whether they are receiving drug A or drug B, it is called single blinding. In this case, researchers are aware of the participant allocation groups.

When the participants as well as the researcher do not know to which treatment group the participants are allocated, it is called double-blinding. In addition to the participants and researcher, if the statistical analyst is also unaware of the allocation, it is called triple blinding. This step-wise blinding from single to double to triple level eliminates subjectivity in the ascertainment of outcomes in a large number of instances. We also need to ensure that the treatments given are identical in terms of colour, appearance and consistency, in addition to blinding for quality control.

7.8 PHASES IN CLINICAL TRIALS AND OBJECTIVES

Typically, all clinical trials are conducted in four phases.

7.8.1 Phase I

The clinical evaluation of any new intervention begins with a trial that is conducted amongst a small number of healthy volunteers (adults/children, men/women), usually below 50 years of age. The goal of this trial is to evaluate if the new intervention is **safe** and **acceptable**.

7.8.2 Phase II

Once the new intervention is found to be safe and acceptable, the clinical trial is moved to phase II. In this phase, the trial is conducted on a larger group, usually comprising 100 to 500 participants. People who are at low risk of acquiring the particular disease are chosen as participants for this phase. The primary aim of this phase is to evaluate the long-term safety, appropriate dose and schedule in case of a vaccine, and identify any early indications of efficacy.

7.8.3 Phase III

Phase III of a clinical trial is a much larger trial that examines the **effectiveness** of a particular intervention under controlled clinical conditions. Generally, these trials involve thousands of individuals who are at high risk of acquiring a particular disease or who are suffering from a particular disease. In a therapeutic scenario, clinical trials help to study how a new drug is effective in curing a disease and in a prevention scenario, they help to evaluate how a prevention measure helps in preventing the occurrence of a disease.

Once phases I, II and III are completed, the product is sent for licensing. After licensing, the new drug is marketed in the country.

7.8.4 Phase IV

Post-marketing surveillance is done in phase IV of clinical trials. This is done on 1000 or more individuals to collect information about the new drug implementation. It is done in a community-based manner rather than in a controlled setting.

All these four phases are integral components of clinical trials.

7.9 EXAMPLES

The following is an example of a '**therapeutic trial**'.

Currently, there is a standard Highly Active Anti-Retro Viral Therapy (HAART) for the treatment of AIDS patients. The treatment consists of three drugs distributed through Anti-Retro Viral Therapy (ART) centres under India's National AIDS Control Programme (NACP).

A researcher wants to study the effect of a New Drug Regimen (NDR) in lowering the viral load and improving CD4 counts in HIV-infected persons. Besides, the researcher believes that the NDR has lesser adverse effects, is cheaper and that the number of tablets to be taken is lesser than in the standard HAART regimen. The researcher wants to evaluate whether this is an optimum regimen that can be used to replace the HAART regiment throughout the country.

To do this, the researcher will first identify HIV-infected individuals and define the inclusion and exclusion criteria for participation. Then, the selected individuals' eligibility for receiving the antiretroviral therapy will be evaluated. The individuals who pass the eligibility screening will be randomised into two groups or arms. One arm will receive the NDR while the other arm will receive the gold standard treatment that is currently available, i.e., HAART. Both the arms will be followed up periodically every six months for the study period of two years. The results of this clinical trial will give the researcher an idea of whether the NDR has worked effectively, and whether there is a difference between the two regimens in lowering the viral load and improving the CD4 count in the two groups. The results will be analysed statistically to determine if NDR is truly beneficial over HAART.

The following is an example of a '**prevention trial**'.

A new vaccine has been developed against the Rotavirus. Sufficient evidence is available from animal studies, supporting safety and the vaccine's ability to generate an immune response against the Rotavirus. It is being considered a promising vaccine for the prevention of Rotavirus disease.

To test if this vaccine can indeed be used to prevent the Rotavirus disease, we will first decide at the national, regional and local level whether this vaccine is appropriate for the country and the population. Then, we will develop a **phase I** trial design for the vaccine. Next, we will find healthy children for recruitment into the study. All the participants will be screened for eligibility and those willing to participate in the study will be randomised into two groups. One group will receive the vaccine, while the other group will receive a placebo. The participants will be followed up periodically for safety assessment.

In clinical trials, safety evaluation is done to document immediate, short-term and long-term adverse effects, usually for 12 to 18 months. The adverse events in both groups will be reported and compared. In addition, serological tests will be conducted to evaluate the participants' immunogenic response to the vaccine. The difference in effects and immunogenicity between the groups will be assessed using statistical methods. This is an example of a prevention trial.

7.10 ADVANTAGES AND DISADVANTAGES OF RCTS

Although clinical trials have certain impediments, they are the only means to make progress in medical science. If there are no clinical trials, no new drugs will be discovered; no new technologies will be invented; no new vaccines will be tested. Hence RCTs must be supported, and adequate information about clinical trials must be disseminated.

7.10.1 Advantages

RCT is the only effective method known to control the selection bias of participants. It also controls confounding bias without any adjustment. Effective blinding is possible. It also has other advantages similar to a cohort or a prospective study.

7.10.2 Disadvantages

Clinical trials involve complex procedures. They require thorough training of all the personnel involved in the trial. They are expensive and often lack representativeness as the volunteers may differ in characteristics from the population of interest, posing a threat to generalisability. They face immense ethical challenges.

Randomised controlled trials are rigorous and difficult to conduct. Yet, progress in medicine and public health is highly unlikely without testing new drugs, therapies, technologies and interventions through trials. Hence, they are considered the gold standard for study designs and are used to generate a high level of evidence to guide decision-making.

References and Further Reading

1. Chapter 4 - Experimental studies and clinical trials. In: World Health Organization. Health research methodology: a guide for training in research methods. Manila: WHO Regional Office for the Western Pacific; 2001: p. 55-70. https://apps.who.int/iris/handle/10665/206929

2. Day SJ, Altman DG. Blinding in clinical trials and other studies. BMJ 2000;321:504. https://www.ncbi.nlm.nih.gov/pmc/articles/PMC1118396/
3. Viera AJ, Bangdiwala SI. Eliminating bias in randomized controlled trials: importance of allocation concealment and masking. Fam Med 2007;39(2):132-7. https://fammedarchives.blob.core.windows.net/imagesandpdfs/fmhub/fm2007/February/Anthony132.pdf

VALIDITY OF EPIDEMIOLOGICAL STUDIES

Tarun Bhatnagar

Learning Objectives

At the end of this chapter, readers will be able to:

1. Discuss the various errors of measurement in epidemiological studies
2. Distinguish between terminologies in epidemiology, such as chance, bias and confounding
3. Identify measures to alleviate the errors of measurement in epidemiological studies

Suppose you come across a newspaper headline: "Coffee Consumption Doubles the Risk of Heart Attack". As a researcher, what would your reaction be? To decide whether to believe this theory or not, you need to know how the study was conducted and how valid its results are.

8.1 OBJECTIVES OF EPIDEMIOLOGICAL STUDIES

The fundamental goal of epidemiological studies is to obtain an accurate estimate of what is being studied—the frequency of a disease or the effect of an exposure on a health outcome. Researchers study these estimates in a sample of the population. **Internal validity** refers to the validity of the methodology that was used to estimate the frequency or determine the effect of an exposure on an outcome. Eventually, the researchers would also want to know whether the estimates are generalisable to the relevant target population among whom the study was conducted. This is known as **external validity**, which indicates the extent to which the research results can be extrapolated to the whole population.

8.2 ACCURACY

Accuracy refers to two things—precision and validity. Let us assume that a person is playing darts. To achieve the best possible result, the player will try to hit the bull's eye as many times as possible. Hitting the bull's eye denotes '**validity**', that is, the extent to which a test measures what it intends to measure. Hitting the bull's eye as many times as possible denotes '**precision**', that is, the proximity of the estimates to the true value.

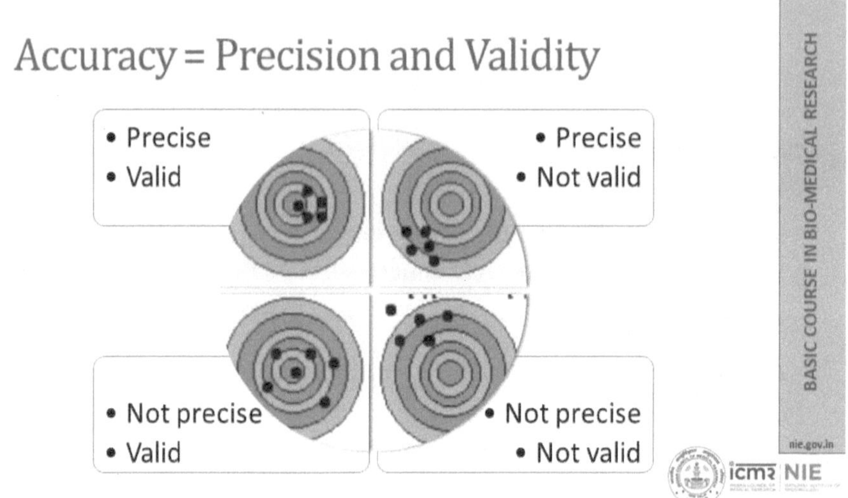

▲ **Figure 8.1:** Depiction of precision and validity in epidemiological studies

Ideally, every epidemiological study must have precise and valid results. However, there can be studies in which the results may be precise, but the methodology may be incorrect. This means that every time researchers conduct that study, they will get similar results. However, the results may not be valid. In contrast, there may be times when the results would be valid but not precise. In a worst-case scenario, the results may neither be precise nor valid. Therefore, researchers should be wary of both precision and validity while interpreting epidemiological studies.

8.3 ERRORS IN ESTIMATION

In epidemiological studies, researchers estimate the frequency of a disease, the health outcome or the effect of an exposure on an outcome. However, these estimates are error-bound. Errors in epidemiological studies are broadly classified as random errors and systematic errors. **Random errors** occur due to chance. These are the variations caused by unknown or uncontrollable factors such as errors in sampling or errors in measurements. The more challenging errors that researchers face are **systematic errors** or **biases**. These are the errors that pose a threat to the validity of any epidemiological study. These errors happen when the methodology used in a study is faulty. If a study is conducted incorrectly, it could produce results far from the truth, thereby leading to errors called **biases**. Ultimately, the results that contain any type of error may differ from the true causal association between the same exposure and outcome in the source population.

Three kinds of biases can occur in any epidemiological study. They are: **selection bias**, **information bias** and **confounding**.

8.4 SELECTION BIAS

Remember that in an epidemiological study, we sample a certain number of individuals to participate in the study. Selection bias can occur in the procedures used to select the study participants from the target population. Researchers need to ensure that the selected study participants actually and accurately represent the target population. Any flaws in selecting a sample from the source population could result in selection bias.

8.4.1 Selection Bias in Case-Control Studies

Let us take the example of a case-control study. In a case-control study, cases and controls are chosen through a surveillance mechanism that provides a systematic notification of cases. If a researcher recruits more exposed cases from the surveillance mechanism, it will result in selection bias. The chances of researchers systematically screening and diagnosing for a particular disease among the exposed are higher if their exposure history is known beforehand. This can again introduce bias artificially. Selection bias can also occur if researchers select cases and controls from healthcare facilities or hospitals, as it is likely that more exposed cases are admitted to these facilities. Selection bias can also occur when researchers select live cases. In this scenario, the patients who died due to the disease would not be a part of the study. The live cases might have survived due to their exposure status, and hence, selection of survived patients can lead to selection bias.

8.4.2 Selection Bias in Cohort Studies

In cohort studies, the participants are followed up over time, and selection bias usually occurs when there is a loss of follow-up. People who are more or less exposed are likely to be lost to follow-up. This can eventually lead to biased results that can be attributed to selection bias.

8.4.3 Addressing Selection Bias

Selection bias can be addressed at any stage of the study—design, data collection or analysis.

- **Design Stage:** Ideally, researchers should ensure that the study is free from selection bias at the design stage itself. One way to confirm this is to use incident cases and not prevalent cases because prevalent cases carry the issue of survival bias. Case-control studies, in particular, are more prone to selection bias; one way of dealing with this is to use a population-based study design rather than a hospital-based design. Researchers can select cases and controls from the community or the population instead of healthcare facilities. Researchers should refrain from leaning towards a particular exposure while selecting cases and controls. Both cases and controls should undergo the same diagnostic procedures with the same intensity of surveillance to prevent any bias at the time of selection.
- **Data Collection Stage:** At the time of data collection, researchers should minimise non-response and non-participation. They should ensure that participants are not lost during follow-up, especially in the case of cohort studies, which have a long follow-up period. They should anticipate loss of participants and document such losses with at least some baseline information such as socio-demographic characteristics. During the analysis stage, researchers can compare the baseline characteristics of the people who were lost to follow-up with that of those who remain in the study to identify any major differences between these two populations that may lead to selection bias. At the time of data collection, researchers should ensure that disease diagnosis is not affected by knowledge about the exposure status. The person who selects cases and controls must not be aware of the participants' exposure status. This method of eliminating selection bias is called blinding.
- **Analysis Stage:** At the analysis stage, the researcher can compare the baseline variables of the participants who responded with that of those who did not respond, or those who dropped out with those who remained in

the study and check if any major or minor differences exist between these two groups. Major or significant differences are suggestive of selection bias. Minor differences could also indicate selection bias, so researchers need to be wary of this. Another way of assessing a selection bias in a study is to conduct a sensitivity analysis. This can give an idea of how bias affects the study results. In sensitivity analysis, the study results and the external information are analysed to deduce the direction and magnitude of bias. If the results are significantly affected, we can assume that selection bias has occurred.

8.5 INFORMATION BIAS

Information bias can occur when researchers measure the characteristics of study participants, such as their exposures, outcomes and other variables. The exposure levels and the presence or absence of an outcome have to be accurately measured. Other variables, referred to as covariates, such as age, gender, education, income, etc., should also be appropriately measured. Researchers should ensure that the measurements taken in the study represent the actual measurements accurately. If a researcher systematically collects information supporting their expected conclusions (consciously or unconsciously), it can lead to information bias. This can be verified during the analysis. In observational epidemiological studies, researchers are dependent on what their study participants tell them; therefore, if there is any systematic distortion of the facts (prevarication) by the study participants, it can result in information bias.

8.5.1 Information Bias in Case-Control Studies

In case-control studies, information bias can occur when researchers collect exposure information inclining towards a particular exposure status. For example, if a researcher collects more information about exposed participants than about unexposed persons or vice versa, it can lead to information bias. Selective recall of the exposure status can also lead to information bias. For example, a researcher asks cases and controls to recall their history of exposures. People who are diseased or have a particular health issue are more likely to recall certain exposures than those who are healthy. This is called **recall bias**. Thus, better exposure data may be available for cases compared to controls, leading to information bias.

8.5.2 Information Bias in Cohort Studies

In cohort studies, information bias can occur when researchers collect information inclining towards a specific outcome status. Thus, if researchers follow the exposed population more rigorously than they do the unexposed population, it can lead to information bias. Besides, better outcome data may be available for the exposed compared to the unexposed, which can also result in information bias.

8.5.3 Addressing Information Bias

For measuring the exposure, outcome and other variables, researchers should set precise operational definitions of what they intend to measure and how they intend to do it. They should develop detailed measurement protocols about how they intend to measure each of these variables. Sometimes, it is good to do repeated measurements of key variables such as blood pressure. We know that blood pressure can vary from time to time, so we can take more than one measurement and then average those measurement readings to capture the actual blood pressure of a particular individual at a given point in time.

It is essential to ensure that the data collectors are trained, certified and re-certified in implementing the study protocol, standard operating procedures and data collection method. Data audits of the interviewers and data management centres can be conducted to ensure that data was collected, retrieved and stored correctly to minimise information bias. Data cleaning should be done after data collection. This can be done visually by eyeballing the data or using computer programs or software. It is a good practice to re-run all analyses before sending your manuscript for publication, to ensure that there is no possibility of any information bias occurring due to how the analysis was done.

8.6 CONFOUNDING

The term **confounding** is derived from a French word that means confusion of effects. In epidemiological studies, researchers study the effect of exposure on the outcome, i.e., whether the participants were exposed and so may be more likely to acquire the disease or vice versa. Thus, their intention is to know the effect of exposure on a particular outcome. This may not be evident in the presence of a third-factor effect that may influence both the exposure and the outcome. At times, the apparent effect of the exposure of interest can be distorted when the effect of extraneous factors is mixed with the actual exposure effect, resulting in confounding.

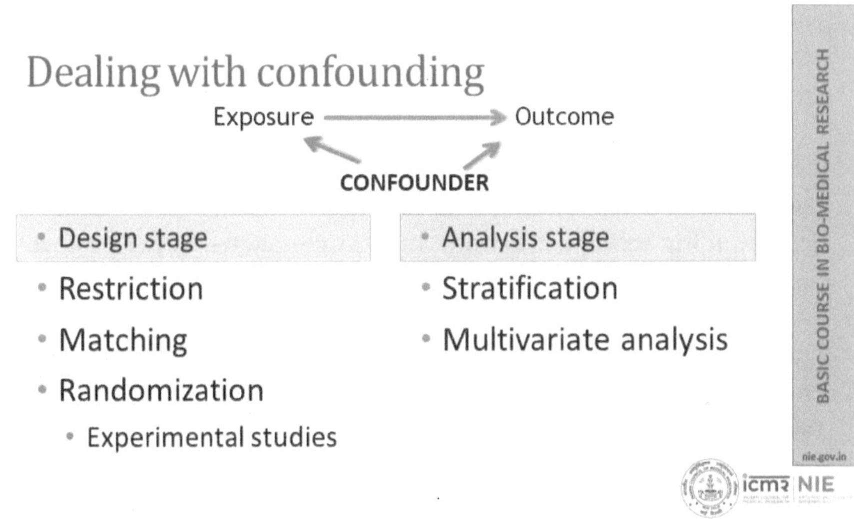

▲ **Figure 8.2:** Relationship of confounder with exposure and outcome

Confounding is one of the biggest threats to the validity of epidemiological studies. Confounding can simulate and show an association that does not exist. It may also hide an association that exists or increase or decrease the strength of the association. In the presence of confounding, researchers may wrongly interpret that the exposure is more associated with the outcome or less associated with the outcome than it actually is. In the worst-case scenario, confounding can also change the direction of an effect. If an exposure causes an outcome due to the influence of confounding, researchers may wrongly infer that the exposure is preventing the occurrence of the outcome. This is the most dangerous threat to validity in any epidemiological study.

8.6.1 Addressing Confounding

Confounding can be addressed both at the design stage and at the analysis stage. However, it is ideal to address it early at the design stage rather than later at the analysis stage.

- **Design Stage:** At the design stage, confounding can be minimised through restriction, matching or randomisation. Restriction means that, researchers can restrict the study participants to only those who are in one stratum of the confounder, so as to avoid the confounder from influencing the association between the exposure and the outcome. Matching means that, if the potential confounders in a particular study are known, the researcher can match cases and controls on those known confounders, to negate their effect. The association between the exposure and outcome thus obtained would be without the influence of the confounder. A matched analysis should be appropriately conducted if matching is done at the design stage of a study. In experimental studies, randomisation is done. Randomisation takes care of confounders and ensures that the two arms in a randomised trial are similar in all ways in terms of the confounding variable, when the study is conducted as per protocol and with adequate sample size.

- **Analysis Stage:** At the analysis stage, stratification and multivariate analysis can be done to identify and address confounding. In statistical analysis, researchers test the data to identify whether there is any confounding and then address it. In stratified analysis, researchers stratify the data into various strata of the confounder and conduct tests of significance to look for any association. This will help in identifying the presence of confounding. Another method of addressing confounding at the analysis stage is using multivariate analysis. In multivariate analysis, researchers use regression techniques such as logistic regression, linear regression or other advanced methodologies to take into account the effect of confounding. The association between the exposure and outcome thus obtained would be without the influence of the confounder or, in other words, adjusted for confounders.

8.7 EVALUATING ASSOCIATIONS BETWEEN EXPOSURE AND OUTCOME

Risk ratio and odds ratio are the standard measures of association between exposure and outcome. An initial analysis between a particular exposure and outcome provides a measure of crude association. Researchers should know to differentiate and identify whether this crude association is actually a true association or a causal association, i.e., whether it represents the true relationship between the exposure and the outcome or not. In order to know this, researchers should work through the process depicted in Figure 8.3 below.

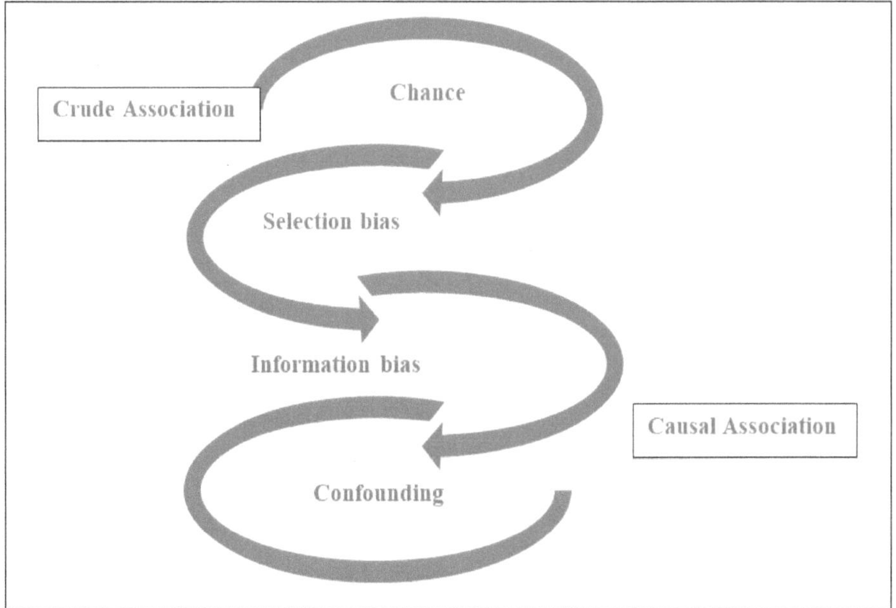

▲ **Figure 8.3:** Steps in evaluating the association between exposure and outcome

As per the spiral shown in Figure 8.3, first, the researchers should rule out the role of chance (based on the p-value for the particular test of significance) when checking for association between an exposure and the outcome of interest. Second, they need to ensure that there is no selection bias. Third, they need to check for any information bias. Fourth, they need to rule out the possibility of confounding and whether that confounding has been appropriately addressed if present. Only after going through this process can one comment on whether the crude association is essentially a causal association or not.

8.8 DOES COFFEE INCREASE THE RISK OF A HEART ATTACK?

At the beginning of this chapter, we discussed a headline in a newspaper: "Coffee Consumption Doubles the Risk of Heart Attack".

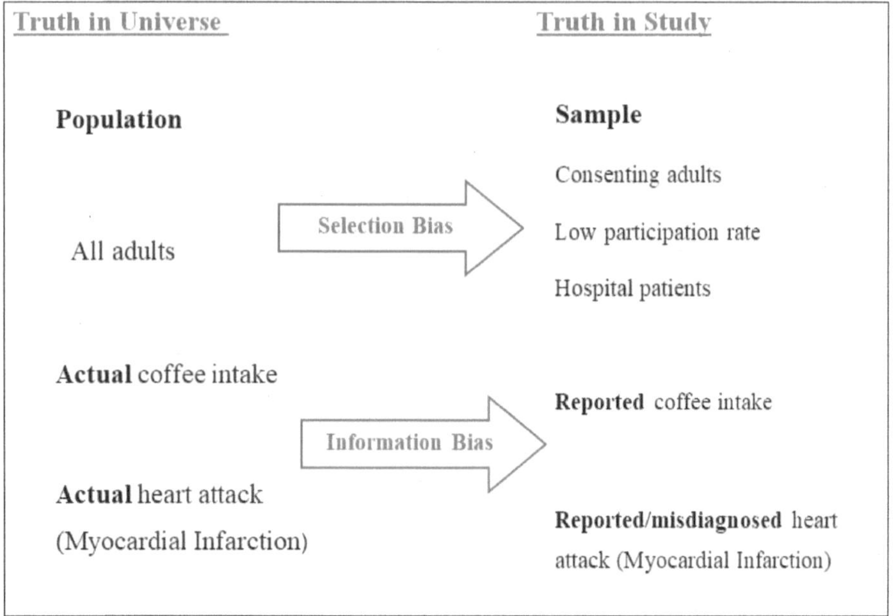

▲ **Figure 8.4:** Schematic representation of bias in a study on the correlation between coffee-drinking and heart attack

A researcher wanted to know if coffee drinkers were at a higher risk of suffering a heart attack than non-drinkers. A sample of individuals who had agreed to participate in the study was chosen. The sample may contain individuals who are more likely to drink coffee as well as individuals who are less likely to drink coffee. If the researcher conducts the study in a hospital setting, these individuals may be hospitalised patients. They may be hospitalised for a condition, say, gastric ulcer, which could have been triggered by coffee-drinking. Thus, the way in which the researcher selects the participants can lead to a bias called selection bias, as discussed earlier.

Here, the exposure of interest is the actual coffee intake of the study participants. However, while collecting data, the researcher obtains this information solely based on what the respondents report. The researcher may have several doubts about the reported coffee drinking: Are the participants reporting their true coffee intake? Do they, in fact, remember how many cups of coffee they have had in the past? What is the average amount of coffee they drink? Do they drink their coffee with milk or without milk? How strong do they take their coffee? These issues can influence whether the coffee intake that the researcher measures is the actual coffee intake or not, which can lead to information bias. The researcher also wanted to know whether the individuals truly had a heart attack or not. It is possible that some patients may have been misdiagnosed with heart attack without adequately ruling out other causes for chest pain. If all cases of chest pain were reported as heart attack, then the study results may be attributed to incorrect assessment, resulting in information bias.

And then, there is confounding. The association between drinking coffee and getting a heart attack may have been confounded by smoking. It is well-established that smoking is a known risk factor for heart attack and that smokers are more prone to heart attacks. It is also known that smokers are more likely to be coffee drinkers. It is possible that since there are more smokers among coffee drinkers and more smokers among those who suffer a heart attack, the association between coffee drinking and heart attack was not due to coffee but because of the effect of smoking. So, the results of the association between drinking coffee (exposure) and having a heart attack (outcome) could have been confounded by the effect of smoking.

8.9 THREATS TO VALIDITY IN EPIDEMIOLOGICAL STUDIES

Researchers must bear in mind that in any epidemiological study, there are various threats to validity that need to be identified and addressed. Biases can occur in all epidemiological studies, more so in observational studies such as case-control and cohort studies and less so in randomised trials. Biases can occur in all stages of the study. If the study is not designed, conducted or analysed properly, it will lead to bias. Biases threaten both internal and external validity. A study with no internal validity cannot be generalised, so it would not have external validity. While designing a study, researchers must think of all possible biases and design the study appropriately to minimise such biases. However, there can be some unavoidable biases. During data analysis, researchers should consider all possible biases and address them wherever possible, and mention those that cannot be addressed as limitations of the study.

References and Further Reading

1. Delgado-Rodri̇guez M, LIorca J. Bias. J Epidemiol Community Health 2004;58:635-41. https://www.ncbi.nlm.nih.gov/pmc/articles/PMC1732856/pdf/v058p00635.pdf
2. Catalogue of bias. https://catalogofbias.org/
3. Zaccai JH. How to assess epidemiological studies. Postgrad Med J 2004;80(941):140-7. https://pubmed.ncbi.nlm.nih.gov/15016934/

QUALITATIVE RESEARCH METHODS: AN OVERVIEW

Tarun Bhatnagar

Learning Objectives

At the end of this chapter, readers will be able to:

1. Recognise the difference between qualitative and quantitative research methods
2. Relate the basic concepts of qualitative research
3. Describe the methods of data management in qualitative research

This chapter is intended to give readers a snapshot of another method of conducting research, called qualitative research methods. In the paradigm of health research or any research, we divide research methods into quantitative and qualitative techniques. Qualitative methods find their origin in the sciences of anthropology, sociology and psychology, which deal with human beings and understanding their behaviours. They are concerned with words/text, unlike quantitative methods that are concerned with numbers.

9.1 DIFFERENCE BETWEEN QUALITATIVE RESEARCH AND QUANTITATIVE RESEARCH

In qualitative research, researchers try to interpret social reality from participants' point of view and experience, rather than measuring it objectively from their own experience; this is known as the '**emic perspective**'. On the other hand, in quantitative research, researchers measure the entities objectively from their own point of view; this is known as the '**etic perspective**'. In terms of logic of inquiry, qualitative methods are inductive, wherein researchers understand social processes through the data collected. In contrast, quantitative methods are deductive, wherein the researchers test their formal hypothesis using the data collected. In terms of research design, qualitative methods involve interpreting the participants' responses rather than presenting the researcher's perspective. On the other hand, quantitative methods ensure repeatability of data; i.e., if somebody else uses the same study methods, they could get similar results.

In qualitative methods, the validity of the results depends on the credibility of the responses collected from the respondents and the credibility of the investigator who conducts the research. In terms of generalisation, qualitative data is more abstract and transcends cultural boundaries. Researchers can understand different cultures from the participants' perspective. Whereas in quantitative methods, more or less the same methodology is applied to understand different cultures.

9.2 USING QUALITATIVE RESEARCH METHODS

Researchers use qualitative research methods to find the answers to a number of questions such as why a particular event happened, how it happened, what were the circumstances that made it happen, why is a health phenomenon occurring and so on. In simple terms, researchers employ qualitative research to gain insight and understand why people behave in a certain way. Qualitative research methods help researchers understand subject matters that are insufficiently researched. When researchers venture into new geographic areas, they need to understand the vocabulary of the region. This is another area where qualitative research could be employed. In social sciences, qualitative research methods help us to view social phenomena more holistically in terms of how participants see them through their eyes.

9.3 RESEARCH METHODS EMPLOYED IN QUALITATIVE RESEARCH

The research methods employed in qualitative research are different from those used in quantitative research. In qualitative research, the methods employed are more interpretative and open-ended. They are more iterative than fixed. The methodology evolves as the research proceeds on, rather than following a pre-structured format. In fact, qualitative research methods foster a partnership between participants and researchers. The researcher becomes an instrument in the research process and acts as a co-interpreter who conveys what the participant wants to say. The main research methods that we use in qualitative research are in-depth interviews, focus group discussions and participant observations.

9.3.1 In-Depth Interviews

In-depth interviews are open-ended interviews that are conducted one-to-one between the researcher and the participant. They are conducted to discover the interviewees' perspective of what they mean in their language. They are also conducted to obtain rich, contextualised and in-depth information. In in-depth interviews, the investigators avoid imposing their structures and assumptions over what the participants want to see.

Technique

In in-depth interviews, interview guides are used to obtain information from the participants. Interview guides are open-ended and unstructured materials that provide guidance regarding the kind of information to be collected from the interviewees. Researchers collect the respondents' perspectives on the topic of interest and use probes to gain a more in-depth understanding of the responses. They then reflect on the remarks made by the respondents. The data thus collected would be in the form of words/text, which would then be recorded or noted down by the researcher. The structure of the information collected and the way the interview takes shape will vary depending on the response given by the participants. Therefore, this is more of an emergent kind of methodology rather than a fixed, pre-structured method.

Using In-Depth Interviews

In-depth interviews are the method of choice when the subject matter is complex and researchers want to know more about it from the respondents. They are also used when the respondents are more knowledgeable about the topic of interest. In-depth interviews are appropriate for highly sensitive subject matters such as sexual behaviours, family planning issues, drug abuse, alcoholism, etc. In-depth interviews are a good way to interact more freely and get more in-depth information from the participants. It comes in handy when the participants are geographically dispersed. In such circumstances, the researchers can talk to them one by one at different times and places to get more information. This technique can also be employed when peer pressure on the respondent is an issue and social desirability is a threat.

Advantages

In-depth interviews, as the name implies, are comprehensive and thorough in nature. Using this technique, researchers can understand why some individuals practice certain behaviours while some do not. It helps gather data on how people think, how they conceptualise their own behaviour and the context in which they do so. In in-depth interviews, the exact words and language used by the participants about the subject matter can be recorded. This gives the researchers an insider's or emic perspective of the subject matter.

Disadvantages

The sampling technique used in in-depth interviews is convenient and purposeful and hence the findings cannot be generalised to the entire population. Unlike quantitative methods in which data is collected on a large number of participants, here, the interviews are conducted among a few knowledgeable participants only. This makes the findings from these interviews not generalisable in the strict quantitative sense. These interviews take a long time; they usually last anywhere between 30 to 45 minutes or may even go beyond an hour. Researchers gather a lot of data in the process, which amounts to a lot of words or textual information. It can be time-consuming to analyse these words. Since the analysis is more interpretative in qualitative research, there is a possibility that the interpretation might turn out how the researcher feels or puts forth the idea in the etic perspective rather than how the participant may have wanted it to be conveyed in the emic perspective.

9.3.2 Focus Group Discussions (FGDs)

Another commonly used method in qualitative research is focus group discussion (FGD). These are open-ended group interviews in which instead of individuals, a small group of people discuss a certain topic among themselves. Usually, six to eight participants who form a homogeneous group in terms of various characteristics like age, gender, socio-economic status, education, occupation, similar cognitive structures and perceptions of their social environment or normative beliefs are chosen. This ensures that the discussion progresses in a cohesive manner.

Technique

In an FGD, there is a moderator who facilitates the whole discussion. Another individual plays the role of a note-taker and takes notes of the topic that is being discussed. Researchers can also make video or audio recordings of these FGDs, to be analysed later on. Similar to in-depth interviews, researchers use an interview guide (topic guide), which contains a list of topics that need to be discussed by the participants in the FGD. The moderator directs the inquiry and ensures that all the topics are discussed as per the researcher's requirements. Interview guides are flexible, in the sense that researchers do not have to strictly follow the chronological order of the questions listed in the guide. It basically flows as per the direction of the ensuing discussion. The moderator should be able to guide the discussion in such a way as to obtain maximum information within the allotted time.

Using FGDs

FGDs are used when group interactions are expected to provide researchers a lot of rich information. In situations where cost and time are constraints, FGDs can be used, as researchers can gather information from more participants in lesser duration of time as compared to in-depth interviews. FGDs help researchers to generate varied ideas from different participants who put forth their ideas from different perspectives. This helps to identify problems and define goals. FGD can be an effective tool for understanding local terminologies and vocabulary. It can also be used to evaluate awareness messages to be used in public health interventions.

Advantages

Some people are more comfortable to talk openly in group settings. In some cultures, this may be a natural way to talk about their problems and personal issues. It is, therefore, a good way to collect information on social norms where people can discuss these issues among themselves. As discussed earlier, FGDs aid the collection of a lot of data in a limited amount of time compared to in-depth interviews.

Disadvantages

Since researchers talk only to a specific group of people, the data that is generated will depend on the actual makeup of this group. Also, when using this methodology, it can be difficult to assess the practice of some very personal or sensitive behaviour. Individuals may be hesitant to talk about sensitive topics in groups. As only a few people participate in FGDs, the data may not be generalisable to the larger target population. The information that researchers gather can be the opinions of vocal and dominant personalities and hence sensitive to biased analysis. Similar to in-depth interviews, FGDs also generate a large amount of data. Many times, it runs into pages, and so transcribing this can be time-consuming. It might be difficult to identify speakers based on the transcript. Hence, it is challenging to analyse this data.

9.3.3 Participant Observation

Another common method that is used in qualitative research is participant observation. This method has its origin in ethnography and anthropology. In this method, the researcher becomes a participant in a social event or the group under study and records his/her observations. The major advantage of this method of research is that researchers get very deep and detailed data because they are a part of whatever is happening in the group. However, one major challenge of this method is that it is sometimes difficult to collect the data systematically. Since the researcher is present in the group, it may be hard to take notes or record the happenings then and there. A few details may hence be forgotten. Analytical methods for participant observation are still evolving; these can again be a challenge in terms of analysis.

9.4 QUALITATIVE DATA (TEXT) ANALYSIS

There are various ways in which qualitative data can be analysed. In most cases, qualitative data means 'text'. There are two approaches to qualitative data analysis—the grounded theory approach and the content analysis approach. The grounded theory approach includes understanding the data and then developing theories based on that. In content analysis, researchers begin with a theoretical framework and then try to analyse the data to understand the theory. In both these methods, researchers should transcribe the interviews into text and, if required, from the local language into English or the language of interest. In the grounded theory approach, the information gathered is coded into themes and categories. The researchers then look for relationships among the categories. Based on these categories, theoretical models are built and then used to understand the perspective of the participants. In content analysis, a set of codes is created for variables and applied systematically to a set of texts. Variable matrix generated from the texts and codes is used as the unit of analysis. In qualitative research, quotes from interviews are used similar to how tables with data are used in quantitative research. These quotes are used as examples to illustrate the main theme that is generated from the data.

9.5 UTILITY OF QUALITATIVE RESEARCH METHODS

Firstly, qualitative research methods could be used just as a tool to generate ideas, as a preliminary step in developing a quantitative study. For example, a researcher wants to understand why people opt for open defecation. The researcher decides to conduct a survey to understand the reasons. But, to ensure that all reasons for open defecation are included in the questionnaire, the researcher has to conduct a qualitative study *a priori* among the target group. Secondly, qualitative research methods can be used to understand the results of a quantitative study. For example, a researcher has conducted a quantitative study. However, the results are inconclusive and require an in-depth understanding of why they got those results. This is where qualitative methods could come in handy. Thirdly, qualitative research methods can be used as the primary data collection method. Qualitative research can be conducted as a standalone method when the objective of the study is to understand human behaviour and get an in-depth understanding of why people do or do not do certain things. For example, why do some communities practice pre-lacteal feeding?

9.6 TRIANGULATION

No single method, whether quantitative or qualitative, can give a holistic picture of any research topic. The researcher could get different explanations or different results when they use different methods. As a researcher, it is important to avoid systematic biases in data collection and interpretation. Therefore, triangulation is used, which involves understanding the topic of interest from different angles, through different methods, by applying different theories and using different data sources. Triangulation of analysts/theory can also be used to control selective and interpretive biases. Researchers can use multiple methods and cull out learnings based on the degree of convergence of information. They can also use different data sources for the same study to understand the differences brought about by these data sources. They can collate all the collected information to gain a comprehensive understanding of the research topic. When different analysts or theories are used, selective perception and interpretative bias will be controlled. Researchers should remember that no single method can solve the problem of rival explanations.

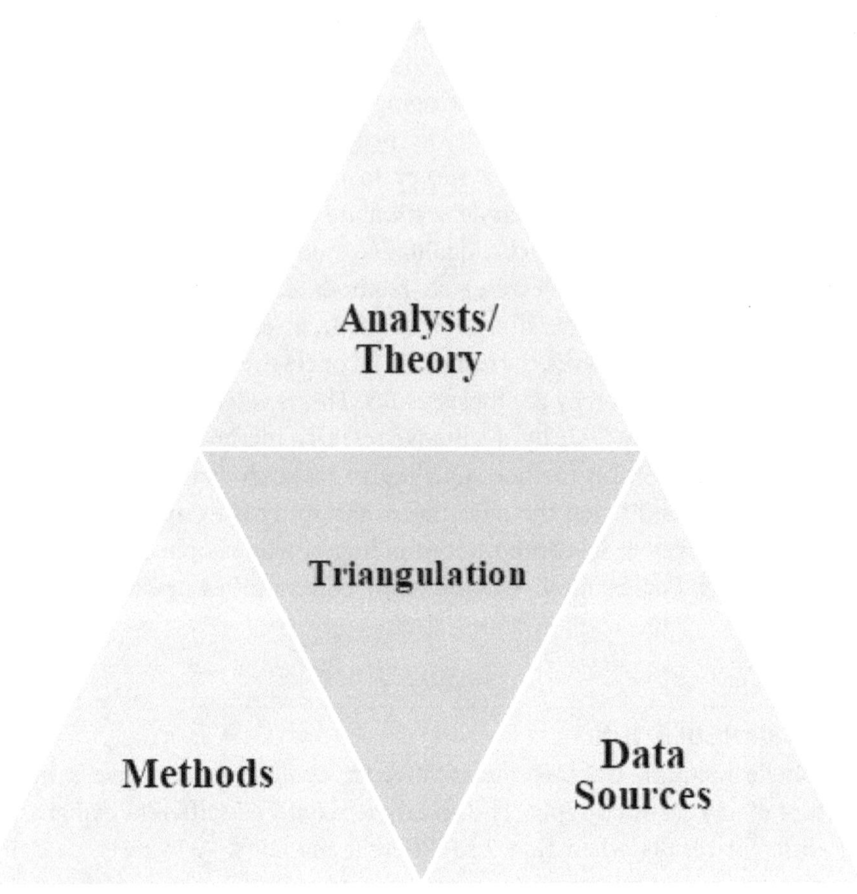

▲ **Figure 9.1:** Methods of triangulation in qualitative research

9.7 HOW ARE QUALITATIVE RESEARCH METHODS USEFUL?

In general, qualitative research methods are useful for identifying the determinants of health. A researcher may ask the following questions: Why do people behave in a certain way? What are their attitudes? What do they perceive about what they are doing or not doing? If interventions were already done, qualitative research methods aid in understanding whether these interventions were successful or not. Qualitative research methods are a good tool to explain social and programmatic impediments to informed choices, such as why people make certain choices or why people use or do not use certain services. These methods are useful for understanding decisions made in the policy, social or legal context.

There are two paradigms in research—qualitative research and quantitative research. Qualitative research is an appropriate way to explore and seek a more in-depth understanding of the topic under study. It is good to use a mix of qualitative and quantitative research methods to get a holistic picture of the research area being studied.

References and Further Reading

1. Hudelson PM. Qualitative research for health programmes. Geneva: World Health Organisation; 2004. http://apps.who.int/iris/bitstream/10665/62315/1/WHO_MNH_PSF_94.3.pdf
2. Tong A, Sainsbury P, Craig J. Consolidated criteria for reporting qualitative research (COREQ): a 32-item checklist for interviews and focus groups. Int J Qual Health Care. 2007;19(6), 349–57. https://academic.oup.com/intqhc/article/19/6/349/1791966
3. Jacob SA, Furgerson SP. Writing interview protocols and conducting interviews: tips for students new to the field of qualitative research. The Qualitative Report2012;17(42):1-10. https://nsuworks.nova.edu/tqr/vol17/iss42/3
4. Ravindran V. Data Analysis in qualitative research. Indian J ContNsgEdn 2019;20(1):40-5. http://www.ijcne.org/article.asp?issn=2230-7354;year=2019;volume=20;issue=1;spage=40;epage=45;aulast=Ravindran

SECTION III

BIO-STATISTICAL CONSIDERATIONS IN DESIGNING A RESEARCH STUDY

MEASUREMENT OF STUDY VARIABLES

R. Ramakrishnan

Learning Objectives

At the end of this chapter, readers will be able to:

1. List the scales of measurement for different types of data
2. Describe and compute the measures of central tendency
3. Explain the purpose of measures of dispersion
4. Illustrate the advantages and disadvantages of these measures

This chapter will discuss data, types of data and how to convert data into information.

10.1 TYPES OF DATA

Data can be broadly classified as qualitative data and quantitative data.

10.1.1 Qualitative Data

Qualitative data refers to a quality or attribute that cannot be quantified. Now, you may wonder, 'what type' of information is qualitative data. Examples of qualitative data include blood groups, such as A/B/AB/O; treatment outcomes, such as cured/not cured/died; colour of the eyes, such as blue/black etc. These are also called categorical variables. Qualitative data could be nominal or ordinal. Nominal data refers to attributes such as the colour of the eyes—blue/brown/black, sex—male/female, regions of the country—north/south/east/west, outcome of a disease—alive/dead etc. Ordinal data refers to information that can be arranged in some order. Example: stages of carcinoma—I/ II/ III, severity of fever—mild/moderate/severe.

10.1.2 Quantitative Data

Quantitative data can be expressed in numbers. It can be divided into two categories: discrete data and continuous data. Discrete data can be counted in whole numbers only. Example: number of siblings, family size. Continuous data can be measured in decimals. Example: height and weight.

10.2 MEASURES OF CENTRAL TENDENCY

Data is used to produce information. However, even if we have huge amounts of data, we cannot get any information just by looking at the data. For this, we need to summarise the data. One of the ways of summarising data is to calculate an average or central tendency. The standard measures of central tendency are:

1. Arithmetic Mean (AM)
2. Median
3. Mode

Arithmetic Mean (AM)

Mean is the most commonly used measure of central tendency. Arithmetic mean (AM) is the most common 'mean' used in the healthcare field. To calculate arithmetic mean, we should add all the observed values (ΣXi) and divide the sum by the number of observations (n).

$$\textbf{\textit{Mean}}\ (\bar{x}) = \frac{\textit{Sum of the values of all observations}\left(\sum Xi\right)}{\textit{Number of observations}\,(n)}$$

Sample mean is denoted as $\bar{x}$ and population mean is denoted as μ.

For example, the ages of 10 pregnant women visiting an antenatal clinic are 26, 31, 25, 21, 26, 26, 27, 25, 27 and 26 years. We can calculate the mean age of these pregnant women by summing up all the ages—which comes to 260—and dividing it by 10. Therefore, the mean age of the pregnant women who visited the antenatal clinic is 26 years.

If there are extreme values in the dataset, they may skew the mean value and lead to overestimation or underestimation of the true measure of central tendency. Hence, to avoid this problem, the central tendency of datasets that contain extreme values should be expressed in terms of 'median'.

Median

Median is the middle value of a distribution. It divides the distribution into two halves; fifty per cent of the data will fall on either side of the median. It is the appropriate measure of central tendency for datasets that have extreme values.

For example, we have data on the duration of hospital stay of 11 patients—1, 2, 3, 4, 5, 6, 7, 8, 8, 9 and 77 days. The data is arranged in ascending order. Here, the middle value is the sixth observation. Therefore, the median of the dataset is 6. Whereas, the mean for this dataset is 11.8. Here, the median (6) is a more appropriate measure of average than the mean (11.8). If the number of observations in the dataset is even, median is calculated by determining the average of the middle two values.

Mode

Mode is the most frequently observed value that occurs in a dataset. In fact, mode is the only statistic of central tendency that is used for nominal data. There could be multiple modes or no mode in a dataset. In epidemiology, we use mode quite often. In an epidemic curve, mode can be used to represent the peaks of waves of cases with respect to time. By looking at the modal class, the researcher can get an idea of the incubation period of the pathogen.

Let us again take the example of the duration of hospital stay of 11 patients—1, 2, 3, 4, 5, 6, 7, 8, 8, 9 and 77 days. Here, 8 occurs twice in the dataset, which is the maximum time. Hence, the mode of this dataset is 8.

10.3 MEASURES OF DISPERSION

Suppose you are 5 feet and 7 inches tall. You visit a swimming pool, but you do not know how to swim. If the pool manager says that the average depth of the swimming pool is 4 feet, will you feel comfortable stepping into the pool? You jump into the pool and realise that you are drowning. You later find out that the pool was 8 feet deep in the place where you jumped in. The question that you missed asking the pool manager was: Is there variability in the depth of the pool? In some places, the pool was as shallow as 3 feet, while in others, it was as deep as 9 feet!

In any research, it is important for the researcher to measure and report the variability of a continuous variable along with the average values. The measures of variability or dispersion are:

1. Range
2. Inter-quartile range
3. Mean deviation
4. Standard deviation
5. Coefficient of variation

Range

Range is the difference between the minimum and the maximum values of the observations. For example, in a study, there are 10 people of ages 20, 25, 19, 47, 56, 25, 26, 29, 35 and 45 years. Here, the range of the age is 20–56. The advantage of range is that it is a quick and easy indicator of dispersion. The disadvantage is that it is influenced by extreme values in the dataset. For range, we consider only two values—the smallest and the largest values in the dataset; we do not consider any other values in between these two values.

Inter-Quartile Range (IQR)

For finding the inter-quartile range, we must divide the dataset into four quarters. This action, to a large extent, takes care of the problem of extreme values. We will consider only the middle fifty per cent of the values to calculate the IQR. The IQR is the third quartile (Q3) minus the first quartile (Q1) [Q3 - Q1]. The greatest advantage of this method is that extreme values do not affect IQR. The disadvantage is that it covers only the middle 50% of the values and ignores the rest of the values.

Mean Deviation

Another measure of variability is mean deviation from mean. In this method, every data point is subtracted from the mean, and then the average of these mean deviations is calculated to measure the mean deviation from the mean. One of the problems with this method is that some values would be lesser, and some would be greater than the mean. Hence, when we sum up all the mean deviations, the value would be 'zero'. So, the mean deviation from the mean would always be 'zero'. To fix this problem, we ignore the sign, calculate the difference, and then take the average. This is called **absolute mean deviation.** The main advantage of mean deviation is that it is based on all observations in the group. The disadvantage is that it ignores the sign of the difference in the value and is mathematically not rigorous enough to use in statistical analyses.

Standard Deviation

Standard deviation is a measure of variability that is commonly used to overcome the disadvantages of mean deviation. In this method, the difference of each observation from the mean are taken, and instead of ignoring the sign as done while calculating absolute mean deviation, the differences are squared to cancel out the minus (-) sign. Then, the average of the summed squared deviations is taken. This is called **variance.** The standard deviation (SD), denoted as σ, is the square root of the average of the squared deviations of the observations from the arithmetic mean. Standard deviation, together with arithmetic means, is useful for expressing continuous data.

Coefficient of Variation

Another statistical measure of dispersion is the coefficient of variation (CV). Unlike standard deviation, coefficient of variation is devoid of any unit. This measure of variability helps to compare the relative variability of variables with different units. Coefficient of variation is the standard deviation expressed as a percentage of the arithmetic mean (AM).

$$CV = \left(\frac{SD}{AM}\right) * 100$$

Standard deviation and arithmetic mean both have the same unit of measurement. Hence, CV is independent of any unit of measurement. Therefore, it is expressed in terms of percentage.

To describe a dataset in a research study, the researcher has to calculate and report a measure of central tendency and variability as appropriate for the variable and data values. Mean and standard deviation are the most appropriate measures of central tendency and dispersion if there are no extreme values in the dataset. However, if the dataset has extreme values, median and interquartile range would be more appropriate measures of central tendency and variability. Nevertheless, the researcher can use mean and standard deviation for a dataset with extreme values after making data transformations. Such transformations require expert data handling and are beyond the scope of this book. Mode and range are normally used for qualitative variables and time distribution in an epidemic curve.

References and Further Reading

1. Campbell MJ, Swinscow TDV. *Statistics at square one. 11th ed.* Chapter 1 - Data display and summary. United Kingdom: Wiley Blackwell; 2009.
2. Ciliska D, Cullum N, Dicenso A. The fundamentals of quantitative measurement. *Evid Based Nurs.* 1999; 2:100-1.
3. Measurement scales and their summary statistics. *BMJ Evid Based Med.* 2004; 9:164-6.

SAMPLING METHODS

R. Ramakrishnan

Learning Objectives

At the end of this chapter, readers will be able to:

1. Recognise the importance of sampling in research
2. Distinguish between probability and non-probability sampling
3. Discuss the strengths and limitations of different types of sampling

In this chapter, we will discuss sampling methods. Sampling is required when you are dealing with a large population and require quick information.

Resources are an important factor for research. If there are enough resources, the entire population can be studied. However, even if enough resources are available, it is not wise to study the entire population, because population is often huge, and time is one of the major constraints in collecting information from a large population. Even if the researcher employs many people to collect data, there could be a lot of inter-observer variations that could add further errors in the study that cannot be measured. Therefore, conducting sample surveys is often the best way to obtain accurate information about large scale population. Hence, even if your study population is the entire universe, the sample could be selected from small regions.

For example, suppose the Ministry of Health of a country wants to estimate the proportion of elementary school children who have been immunised against childhood infectious diseases in one month. The study population for this survey is large, so it will be difficult to complete the whole survey within one month. In this case, we should estimate the proportion of immunised children by testing a sample of the children who represent the study population.

11.1 DEFINITIONS

Let us now look at the definitions of some of the concepts related to sampling.

11.1.1 Sampling

Sampling is the procedure of selecting some members of the population, who are representative of the entire population. If we have a large number of people and select a portion of them, then it is called sampling.

11.1.2 Study Population

Study population is the population to which the study results are to be inferred.

▼ **Table 11.1:** Examples of research questions and study population

Research question	Study population
How many injections do people receive each year in India?	The entire population of India
How many healthcare workers experience a needle-stick injury each year in India?	Healthcare workers of India
How many hospitals have a needle-stick prevention policy in India?	All hospitals in India

11.1.3 Representativeness

The sampled people should be representative of the population in terms of geographical distribution (such as urban or rural), population characteristics (such as age, sex and demography) and time (such as seasonality and day of the week).

11.1.4 Sampling Unit

These are the elementary units that will be sampled. Sometimes, they are called Basic Sampling Unit (BSU).

For example, in Table 11.1, each of the selected Indians (example 1), healthcare workers (example 2), and hospitals (example 3) comprise the sampling unit.

11.1.5 Sampling Frame

A sampling frame is a list of all the sampling units in a population.

For example, in Table 11.1, a list of all Indians (example 1), all healthcare workers in India (example 2) or all hospitals in India (example 3) will comprise the sampling frame for the relevant research questions.

11.1.6 Sampling Scheme

Sampling scheme is a method used to select sampling units from the sampling frame.

11.1.7 Sampling Error

No sample is a perfect mirror image of the population. When we pick a sample from a population and implement our study in the sampled group, the results may not be the same as the results we would get if we consider the entire population. This type of deviation of the sampled value to the true population estimates is known as **sampling error**. Sampling errors could occur if the sample is not representative of the study population. But fortunately, the magnitude of this error can be measured as probability in the case of random sampling. This is known as the standard error of mean or proportion or differences. Sampling errors can be minimised through random selection of samples or by increasing the sample size. Sampling error is an important component in sampling theory, as it helps in identifying the appropriate sample size.

11.2 TYPES OF SAMPLING

There are different ways in which a population can be sampled. Broadly, sampling is classified into two types: non-probability sampling and probability sampling.

Non-Probability Sampling Methods

i. Convenience Sampling / Purposive Sampling

Probability Sampling Methods

i. Simple Random Sampling
ii. Stratified Random Sampling
iii. Systematic Random Sampling
iv. Cluster Sampling
v. Multistage Sampling

11.2.1 Non-Probability Sampling

Non-probability sampling is a method of selecting samples wherein the probability of the sample being selected for the study is unknown. It could be **convenience sampling** or **purposive sampling**.

i) Convenience Sampling / Purposive Sampling

When researchers choose study participants who are closer to their reach and convenient for them, it is called convenience sampling. For example, a researcher could include the first 100 people that he/she comes across in the study. This is a convenience sample. The disadvantage of this type of sampling is that the sample could be biased; it could either give the best or the worst scenario. Also, as these would be subjective samples, deriving objective criteria from them would be difficult. Nevertheless, non-probability sampling methods are still useful and are being extensively used to generate hypotheses.

11.2.2 Probability Sampling

In the probability sampling method, every unit in the population has a known probability of being selected. This type of sampling allows us to draw valid conclusions about the population. It removes the possibility of bias in the selection of participants and ensures that each subject has a known probability of being chosen. Statistical tests can be applied to probability sampling because most statistical tests are valid only if the samples are drawn randomly.

i) Simple Random Sampling

This is the simplest form of probability sampling. In simple random sampling, every individual unit has an equal chance of being included in the sample.

Procedure

In simple random sampling, all the units in the sampling frame are numbered, and then the required sample units are drawn randomly either by '**lottery**' or using a **table of random numbers.**

For example, suppose we have to choose 4 units from a complete list of 48 items. First, each item is given a number (from 1 to 48), and then these numbers are written on small chits of paper. Then, all the chits are placed in a pile, and by lottery method, 4 chits are chosen randomly, and these numbers are recorded. Let us assume that 9, 18, 32 and 40 are the chosen numbers. The items that were given these numbers would be selected as samples.

Advantages

1. It is simple to perform.
2. Sampling error can be easily measured.

Limitations

1. A complete list of all sampling units should be available before recruiting samples from the population. Many times, this list may not be available.
2. It does not always provide the best representation of the study population. Sometimes, the sampled population may be different from the whole population, and not representative of the population.

ii) Systematic Random Sampling

Systematic random sampling is a type of probability sampling in which samples are selected at regular intervals from a complete list of sampling units.

Procedure

Systematic random sampling is done by randomly selecting the initial sampling unit and then every k^{th} *unit* from the sampling frame. For example, if a sampling frame has a total of N units and n is the sample to be selected from the entire sampling frame, then k, known as the sampling interval, is obtained by dividing the entire population by the sample size (k=N/n). Then, a number less than or equal to k (≤ k) is randomly selected as the first sample. After this, every k^{th} unit from the sampling frame is selected. Therefore, every unit has an equal chance of being selected.

For example, if a systematic random sample of 10 houses is to be selected from a list of 100 houses, the sampling interval, k = 100/10 = 10. Now, we select a number between 1 and 10 randomly. The first house to be included in the sample is chosen by randomly picking one out of ten chits of paper numbered from 1 to 10. Let us assume that the number picked is 8. Hence, the eighth house will be selected first, and then every tenth house will be selected starting from the first selected house, until the desired sample size is achieved.

Advantages

1. This method ensures representativeness across the list.
2. It is easy to implement.

Limitations

1. If there is a cyclical pattern of specific characters within the sampling frame being studied, we might probably draw an atypical sample.
2. Some statistical measures are difficult to compute if the samples are selected through systematic random sampling. In such cases, we do not use the exact formula, but use an approximate form of the formula.

iii) Stratified Random Sampling

The principle of stratified random sampling is to classify the entire population into homogeneous subgroups called **strata**, and draw random or systematic samples of a pre-determined size from each stratum. Then, we combine the results of all these strata to get an idea of the entire population.

For example, suppose we want to estimate the coverage of vaccination in an entire country. To do this, we can divide the country into four regions—East, West, North and South—and draw samples from each of the four regions. We can estimate the vaccination coverage for each stratum separately and calculate the combined coverage for the entire country by weighing each stratum based on the size of the region.

Advantages

1. It is more precise if the outcome of interest is associated with the strata.
2. We can make inferences about subgroups separately as all subgroups are represented in the sample.

Disadvantages

1. It is difficult to measure sampling error in stratified sampling.
2. There could be a loss in precision if the sample includes many strata and each stratum contains small samples.

iv) Cluster Sampling

Another important type of random sampling that is mostly used in health care surveys is cluster sampling. In this type of sampling, a random sample of groups of study units (or clusters) is selected instead of an individual study unit. **Clusters** are mostly geographic units (such as villages, census enumeration blocks, wards, etc.) or institutional units (such as schools, colleges, hospitals, etc.). Here, the sampling unit is not a subject but a group or a cluster of participants. The assumption is that the variability among the clusters is minimal, while the variability within each cluster is what is observed in the general population.

Cluster sampling is generally performed when the population is distributed over a large area and the researcher needs to collect a representative sample from the population using limited resources.

Procedure

Two-stage cluster sampling: Usually, cluster sampling is done in a two-stage approach.

In the **first stage**, a pre-determined number of clusters is selected by applying the principle of **probability proportional to size (PPS)**. This is done by performing the following steps:

a) A cumulative list of all clusters (e.g., villages) in the entire population is prepared and the grand total is computed.

b) The grand total is divided by the number of clusters to obtain the sampling interval.

c) A random number that is less than the sampling interval is chosen and using this number, the first cluster is identified.

d) The sampling interval is added to the first random number to identify the second cluster.

e) This procedure is repeated to identify all other clusters.

In the **second stage**, in each selected cluster, a sampling frame of all members is prepared. From the sampling frame, the desired sample size is selected through simple random sampling or systematic random sampling.

Advantages

1. This method of sampling is simple and does not require a list of all sampling units. Only the list of sampling units in the selected cluster is needed.
2. It is economical. Less travel and resources are required.

Disadvantage

If the clusters are homogeneous, the researcher might end up with a large design. All the people in the sample may have very homogeneous results, resulting in high sampling error, which is difficult to measure in cluster sampling.

v) Multistage Sampling

In the case of a large and diverse population, sampling needs to be done in two or more stages. For example, if we want to conduct a research at the national level, we could divide the samples into several parts like regions (East, West, North and South), then every region into districts and then each district into census enumeration blocks. Lastly, from each block, pre-determined households and desired individuals can be selected.

Advantages

1. Initially, no list of the population is required.
2. It is the most feasible approach for large populations.

Disadvantage

There are several stages of sampling; hence sampling error will be high. Calculation of sampling error is very difficult unless certain specific methodologies are followed for selection at each stage.

When conducting a research, the entire population cannot be included in the study. Therefore, sampling is necessary. Sampling can cause sampling error, but that can be measured. Good study design and quality assurance will help ensure the validity of study findings, while an appropriate sample size will help ensure precision. Probability sampling is the most preferred type of sampling, as it allows the use of statistics and can provide a valid conclusion.

References and Further Reading

1. World Health Organization. *Health research methodology: a guide for training in research methods*. Manila: WHO Regional Office for the Western Pacific; 2001: p.71-83.
2. Elfil M, Negida A. Sampling methods in clinical research: an educational review. *Emerg (Tehran)*. 2017; 5(1): e52.
3. Martínez-Mesa J, González-Chica DA, Duquia RP, Bonamigo RR, Bastos JL. Sampling: how to select participants in my research study? *An Bras Dermatol*. 2016;91(3):326–30.

CALCULATING SAMPLE SIZE AND POWER

R. Ramakrishnan

Learning Objectives

At the end of this chapter, readers will be able to:

1. Recognise the role of sample size and power in a statistical test
2. Outline the steps in estimating a sample size
3. Determine the sample size required to estimate population parameters
4. Describe design effect and its influence on statistical power

The previous chapter discussed the importance of sampling and various sampling strategies. While conducting a research, the researcher should know how many patients need to be recruited for the study from a clinician's perspective. This requires logical thinking, and usually depends on some of the information that the researcher should understand before initiating the study. Therefore, sample size calculation is a very important procedure in conducting a research. This chapter will provide a brief idea about sample size calculation for different study designs.

12.1 IMPORTANT CONCEPTS RELATED TO SAMPLE SIZE CALCULATION

Precision

Precision is an important parameter that plays a significant role in sample size calculation. It refers to how close an estimate is to the actual value of a population parameter. It may be expressed in absolute terms or relative to the forecast. For example, 10% absolute precision is expected in a research study to measure the prevalence of child malnutrition. This means that the estimated prevalence of child malnutrition will be ten percentage points on either side (plus or minus 10%) of the true population parameter. A relative precision of 10% means that the resulting estimated prevalence will fall within 10% (not percentage points) of the true population parameter.

Type I Error

'Type I error' or Alpha (α) error is the level of false-positive error that a researcher can accept in their study during hypothesis testing. It occurs when the researcher rejects a null hypothesis when it is true. When there is a Type 1 error, even if there is no real difference between the two groups, such as the treatment group and the control group in a randomised controlled trial, the researcher can infer that a significant difference in outcome exists between the treatment and the control groups.

Alpha (α) and Confidence Level

Alpha (α) is the probability of rejecting a null hypothesis when it is true. It denotes the significance level of a test. By convention, in health research, an alpha value of 5% or a significance level of 0.05 is often accepted.

Confidence level is the complement of alpha error. It is the probability that an estimate of a population parameter is within certain specified limits of the true value. It is denoted by $1-\alpha$.

Type II Error

Type II error or Beta (β) error is the level of false-negative error that the researcher is willing to accept in their study during hypothesis testing. This type of error occurs when the researcher fails to reject a null hypothesis when it is false. In this case, even if there is a real difference between the two groups, such as the treatment group and the control group in a randomised controlled trial, the researcher has inferred that no significant difference exists in the outcome between the treatment group and the control group.

Beta (β) and Power

Beta (β) error is the probability of failing to reject a null hypothesis when it is false. In other words, it is the probability of committing a Type II error. Power is the probability of correctly rejecting the null hypothesis when it is false. It is denoted as '$1-\beta$'.

12.2 FACTORS USED IN SAMPLE SIZE ESTIMATION

Calculation of sample size depends on the following factors:

- Study variable
- Type of estimate
- Expected frequency of variable of interest
- Desired precision of the estimate
- Acceptable risk that the estimate will fall outside its real population value (alpha level)
- Population size
- Design effect
- Response rate

Study Variable

During the planning stage of a study, the researcher should decide on the primary study variables. For example, if the researcher wants to analyse the magnitude of scrub typhus in a community, the study will aim to estimate the prevalence of scrub typhus. In this case, the primary study variable is whether a person has scrub typhus or not. Suppose the researcher is interested in the factors associated with scrub typhus. Demographic characteristics, occupation, living conditions, sanitation/hygiene practices, seasonality, exposure to domestic animals and rodents, and presence of surrounding shrubs and bushes are the study variables. There may be many variables in a study; the researcher has to identify which variable they want to focus on.

Type of Estimate

The second step is to choose the measure of estimation for the study. Depending on the characteristics of the variable, the researcher can select mean, ratio or proportion. The formulae for computing the sample size will differ based on the type of estimate chosen. For example, the sample size formula will vary based on whether the variable is continuous or categorical.

Expected Frequency of the Variable of Interest

The next factor for calculating sample size is the expected frequency of the variable of interest. For example, a study on a rare disease will need a larger sample size when compared to a study on a common disease. This is because, when the research is on a rare disease, unless a large number of people are observed, adequate data on the event or disease cannot be generated.

Desired Precision

The next important factor for sample size calculation is the desired precision of the estimate. The researcher may want a more precise estimate, such as within 5% of the true value, or a less precise estimate, such as within 10% of the true value. A more accurate estimate will require a larger sample size. Thus, the sample size will increase as the precision of the estimate increases.

Acceptable Risk That Estimate Will Fall Outside Its Real Population Value (Alpha Level)

Another critical parameter in sample size calculation is the maximum amount of risk the researcher is willing to take in interfering with the study result. Usually, researchers accept a 5 per cent risk of making an error while rejecting the null hypothesis.

Adjust for Population Size

Adjustments for population are made during sample size calculation. Researchers should decide whether they will draw the sample from a large or small population because sample size formulae assume that we are drawing a sample from a large population. So, if we draw a sample from a small population, we need to adjust the sample size formulae accordingly.

Design Effect

We discussed the design effect of cluster sampling in the previous chapter, wherein a group of people is selected rather than individuals. In cluster sampling, biases are introduced when the study participants are not independent of each other. Cluster sampling will have some homogeneity with respect to the outcome of interest among the participants in the same cluster. Design effect compensates for the variability present within and among the study participants in a cluster.

Response Rate

Suppose a researcher requires a sample size of 300 participants; it may not be possible to gather the said number of participants during data collection. If there is a 10 per cent loss in the number of study participants than what is required, the researcher has to add an extra 10 per cent to the estimated sample size to adjust for non-response. The sample will then be sufficient to answer the research question even with a non-response.

12.3 SAMPLE SIZE REQUIRED FOR ESTIMATING POPULATION MEAN

Suppose a researcher aims to estimate the mean of a population; the following parameters are required to calculate the sample size:

Z_α = Standard normal deviation (For a 95% confidence interval, the value is taken as 1.96)

SD = Standard deviation

d = Allowable error (also called precision)

Using the equation below, the required sample size 'n' can be calculated.

$$d = Z\,\frac{\sigma}{\sqrt{n}}$$

$$\text{Therefore, } n = \frac{Z^2\sigma^2}{d^2}$$

Example:

A nutritionist wishes to determine the average daily protein intake of teenage girls by conducting a survey. The information required to calculate the sample size for this survey are (i) the desired width of the confidence interval (precision), (ii) the level of confidence desired and (iii) the magnitude of the population variance.

Assume that the nutritionist wants the width of the confidence interval to be 10 units of the expected mean protein intake (i.e., absolute precision of 5 units) and a 95 per cent level of confidence.

The nutritionist estimates the population standard deviation to be about 20 grams by performing a literature review.

Z = 1.96 (For a 95% confidence interval, the standard normal deviation value is taken as 1.96)

SD (σ) = 20

Desired length (d) = 5 units

Let us now substitute the values in the formula to find the value of n.

$$n = \frac{(1.96)^2(20)^2}{(5)^2} = 61.47$$

This means that the nutritionist needs to have a sample size of at least 62 teenage girls in order to get an estimate of the mean protein intake within five units on either side of the true mean population protein intake.

12.4 SAMPLE SIZE REQUIRED FOR ESTIMATING POPULATION PROPORTIONS

In order to estimate a population proportion, researchers must know the anticipated proportion (p) of the variable of interest in the population. Researchers can perform a literature search or conduct a pilot study to get an idea of 'p'. However, if it is impossible to determine the value of p, the best possible approach is to assume a value of p = 0.5, as it will yield the maximum sample size.

To calculate the sample size, the following information are required:

Z_α = Standard normal deviation (For a 95% confidence interval, the value is taken as 1.96)

p = anticipated proportion of the variable of interest

d = Allowable error (also called precision)

The formula is:

$$n = \frac{z^2 p * q}{d^2}, \text{ where } q = 1 - p$$

Example:

A state immunisation officer wants to estimate the actual immunisation coverage in a community of school children. Previous studies found that immunisation coverage should be around 80 per cent. Suppose the immunisation officer would like to measure the result within 4 per cent of the actual value (absolute precision) with a confidence level of 5%.

The values required for the sample size calculation are:

d = absolute precision = 0.04

p = expected proportion in the population = 0.80, q = 0.2

Z_α = 1.96 (for a 5% confidence level)

Therefore,

$$n = \frac{z^2 p * (1 - p)}{d^2}$$

$$= \frac{(1.96)^2 (0.80) * (0.20)}{(0.04)^2} = 384$$

Hence, the immunisation officer needs to include 384 participants in the study to determine an estimate of the immunisation coverage within 4% of either side.

12.5 SAMPLE SIZE CALCULATION FOR ANALYTICAL STUDIES

In the case of analytical studies such as case-control or cohort studies, researchers need to know the desired values of Zα and Zβ, the anticipated proportion of exposure in the study participants with the disease (cases) and participants without the disease (controls) in the case of case-control studies and the expected ratio of illness among exposed and unexposed participants in the case of cohort studies. The required values can be taken from previous studies or reports. Additionally, the magnitude of the expected strength of association in the analyses (odds ratio in a case-control study and risk ratio in a cohort study) is required. These can also be obtained from previous studies or reports.

12.5.1 Sample Size Calculation for Cohort Study

A cohort study was conducted to study the risk of myocardial infarction among women of childbearing age, who were using oral contraceptives (OC). Previous studies have indicated that the proportion of non-OC users at risk of the said disease is 15%. This means that 15% of non-OC using women of childbearing age are at risk of myocardial infarction. The proportion of OC users at risk of the disease is 25%. Suppose the researcher wants to calculate the sample size for the study at a 5% confidence level (α is 0.05) with a power of 80% (β is 0.20). Also, assume that the researcher will use an equal sample size for both groups (users and non-users).

The formula for determining the sample size is as follows:

$$n = \frac{(z_{1-\alpha/2+} z_{1-\beta})^2 \, (p_0 q_0 + p_1 q_1)}{(p_1 - p_0)^2}$$

Here, p_0 is the proportion of non-OC users with the disease = 0.15

p_1 is the proportion of OC users with the disease = 0.25

q_0 (complement of p_0) = 0.85

q_1 (complement of p_1) = 0.75

$Z_{(1-\alpha/2)} = 1.96$ and $Z_{(1-\beta)} = 0.84$

Thus,

$$n = \frac{(z_{1-\alpha/2+} z_{1-\beta})^2 \, (p_0 q_0 + p_1 q_1)}{(p_1 - p_0)^2}$$

$$= \frac{(1.96+0.84)^2 \, (0.15*0.85+0.25*0.75)}{(0.25-0.15)^2}$$

$$= \frac{(0.315)*(7.84)}{0.01} = 246.96 = 247$$

Therefore, a minimum of 247 OC users and 247 non-OC users are required for the cohort study.

12.5.2 Sample Size Calculation for Case-Control Study

A case-control study was conducted to estimate the risk of myocardial infarction among women of childbearing age, who were using oral contraceptives. Previous literature observed that 10 per cent of women use oral contraceptives (OC), and the odds ratio (OR) of myocardial infarction associated with current OC use is 1.8. The researcher considers a 5% confidence level and 80% power for the study. Hence, $\alpha = 0.05$ and $\beta = 0.20$. The study employs an equal size of cases and controls. The required parameters for sample size calculation are:

p_0 = proportion of controls who are current OC users = 0.10
p_1 = proportion of cases who are current OC users = 0.18
$q_0 = 0.9$
$q_1 = 0.82$
$Z_{(1-\alpha/2)} = 1.96$ and $Z_{(1-\beta)} = 0.84$
Therefore, the sample size,

$$n = \frac{(z_{1-\alpha/2+}z_{1-\beta})^2\,(p_0q_0 + p_1q_1)}{(p_{1-}p_0)^2}$$

$$= \frac{(1.96+0.84)^2\,(0.10*0.90+0.18*0.82)}{(0.18-0.10)^2}$$

$$= \frac{(0.2376)*(7.84)}{0.0064} = 291.06 = 292$$

Hence, a minimum of 292 cases and 292 controls are needed for this case-control study.

Further, the required sample size will vary as the magnitude of association (relative risk or odds ratio) changes. For example, to detect an OR of 1.2, a minimum sample size of 3834 is required; whereas, for an OR of 3, a sample size of 59 is enough in each group. This means that a large sample size is required to detect a small difference of effect among groups, and a smaller sample size is required to detect a large difference of effect among groups.

12.5.3 The 10% Rule

In analytical studies, while looking for an association of one variable, the researcher may come across a third factor that could affect the results of this association. This third factor is known as confounder. There could be multiple confounders for an association. It is proposed that for each confounder, 10% of the sample size should be increased.

Thus, no 'magic number' is available for sample size. It has to be computed based on various parameters assumed by the researcher. Researchers should provide references to the assumptions considered in the study and the software used to calculate the sample size in their research report. Free open-source computer applications are available for computing sample sizes for different study designs. For example: OpenEpi (www.openepi.com) can be used for power and sample size calculation. If details about the parameters are not available, the researcher may conduct a pilot study, and values obtained from the pilot study can be used for sample size calculation. These details should be mentioned in the Methods section of the report or manuscript.

References and Further Reading

1. Lwanga SK. Lemeshow S. Sample size determination in health studies - a practical manual. Geneva:World Health Organization; 1991.
2. Hickey GL, Grant SW, Dunning J, Siepe M. Statistical primer: sample size and power calculations—why, when and how? *Eur J CardiothoracSurg.*2018; 54:4–9.
3. Jones SR, Carley S, Harrison M. An introduction to power and sample size estimation. *Emerg Med J.* 2003; 20:453-8.
4. World Health Organization. Health research methodology: a guide for training in research methods. Manila: WHO Regional Office for the Western Pacific; 2001: p.71-83.

SECTION IV

PLANNING A RESEARCH STUDY

SELECTION OF STUDY PARTICIPANTS

P. Ganesh Kumar

Learning Objectives

At the end of this chapter, readers will be able to:

1. State the fundamental principles of project management
2. Describe the road map to study planning and management
3. Recognise the common reasons for study failure

A good choice of study participants serves the vital purpose of ensuring that the findings of the study accurately represent the population of interest. The selection of appropriate study participants who can help gather accurate information about the population of interest is a critical requirement in health research. Researchers should remember three crucial points while selecting study participants from the population of interest.

1. The activity should be completed within an acceptable cost in terms of time and money.
2. The selected size of study participants should be adequate to control random error.
3. The study participants should be representative of the population of interest. If the study participants are representative, the findings can be generalised to the population of interest.

In the previous chapters, we had discussed about various sampling techniques used in research and how to calculate an adequate sample size for different study designs. In this chapter, we will see how to select representative study participants and the issues that can arise when selecting study participants. We will also learn about participant recruitment strategies.

13.1 TERMINOLOGIES RELATED TO STUDY POPULATION AND SAMPLE

The specific terminologies related to study participants that are used in health research are discussed below.

Target Population: Population denotes people living in a large geographical area—for example, the population of India or the population of Tamil Nadu. When a researcher defines specific clinical and demographic characteristics of a large population to demarcate the population of interest for the research, it is known as target population. Target population is a population on which the research findings can be generalised. For every research, the target population has to be clearly defined. The selection of target population should be based on the research question (Figure 13.1).

Accessible Population: Accessible population is the part of the target population who are available and willing to participate in the study. Accessible population can be derived by applying specific geographical, temporal and budgetary criteria to the target population. Therefore, accessible population is a subset of target population (Figure 13.1).

Sample: The study sample is a subset of the accessible population among whom the research is conducted. The study sample consists of the study participants.

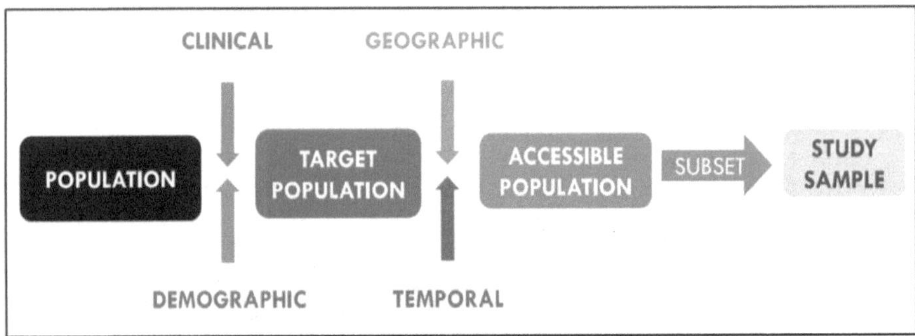

▲ **Figure 13.1:** Selection of study sample from population

13.2 STEPS FOR SELECTING STUDY POPULATION

The steps involved in selecting the study population are listed below (Figure 13.1):

- In the first step, the researcher must define the target population by applying specific inclusion criteria to the population with respect to clinical and demographic characteristics.
- In the second step, the accessible population should be selected by applying a particular set of inclusion criteria to the target population with respect to geographic and temporal characteristics, as decided in the study protocol.
- In the third step, a subset of the accessible population must be selected by applying the exclusion criteria.
- In the fourth step, the estimated sample size must be chosen using an appropriate sampling method. The sample size should be adequate to control random errors in the study.
- Finally, in the fifth step, an appropriate recruitment strategy must be used to recruit representative study participants and facilitate the study's non-response rate.

For example, suppose the research question for a study is, "What is the lowest dose of Metformin that can be given to reduce dysmenorrhea among females having polycystic ovary syndrome (PCOS) in the reproductive age group?" Here, the target population is females in the reproductive age group who suffer from PCOS and have a clinical feature of dysmenorrhea. Thus, the target population is defined using specific clinical (PCOS and dysmenorrhea) and demographic (reproductive age group) characteristics. Adding geographic and temporal characteristics will help the researchers to obtain a subset of the target population known as the accessible population. In this example, if the researcher conducts the study in a particular city and among patients who get treated at a specific clinic or out-patient department (OPD), that will be the accessible population defined using geographic characteristics.

Additionally, if the researcher recruits participants between January 1 to December 31 of a specific year, it will amount to setting the temporal criteria. Therefore, all the females in the reproductive age group with PCOS and dysmenorrhea (clinical and demographic characteristics) getting treated at a specific clinic or OPD from January 1 to December 31 (geographic and temporal characteristics) will be recruited for the study. From this accessible population, as per the estimated sample size, the study sample or study participants will be recruited.

13.3 CHOOSING REPRESENTATIVE STUDY PARTICIPANTS

In choosing representative study participants, two important terminologies need to be understood: 'external validity' and 'internal validity'.

After framing the research question, the target population is identified based on specific clinical and demographic characteristics. Then, the accessible population is selected from the target population and finally, the study participants are chosen from the accessible population.

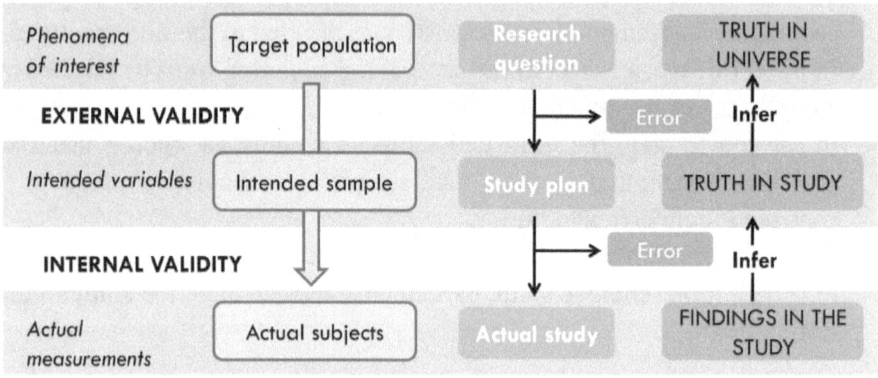

▲ **Figure 13.2:** Implications of the results of a research on study population

Study findings can be inferred after the completion of a research. The study findings inferred directly from the study participants are known as 'truth'. However, researchers always try to extrapolate this truth that applies to the target population as the truth of the universe. They try to generalise their study findings for the target population. However, it should be kept in mind that random errors may occur when selecting participants from the target population. These errors can be addressed by picking an adequate study sample (Figure 13.2).

13.4 INTERNAL VALIDITY AND EXTERNAL VALIDITY

Studies that have good internal validity can be generalised to other populations. However, one has to keep in mind that internally valid results are not necessarily generalisable to the target population. There is always a trade-off between internal validity and generalisation. Generalisability is not a categorical answer of yes or no. Rather, it is a mix of scientific and practical decisions taken when choosing study participants and applying the study findings to the population of interest. Therefore, generalisability depends on the research question, study design and method applied to derive the findings.

Now, what is the internal and external validity of research?

The internal validity of a research is the extent to which the observed results of a study are consistent with the population's truth. Thus, if the study findings are compatible with the true values in the population, then the study is internally valid. Whereas external validity of a study defines to what extent the study's findings are generalisable to the target population and in other study settings or samples. Internal validity is an essential characteristic of research. Only if a study is internally valid, the researcher can think about generalising the interpretation of the study to other populations. If researchers are not choosing representative samples from the population, it means that they are subject to more bias and confounding than the internally valid samples.

Most studies are often generalisable—for example, in the Framingham cohort study, individuals from the Framingham county were selected as the study population. Now, the question is whether the findings of this study can be generalised to the whole population of the United States of America. This study found that the strength of association between cardiovascular diseases and risk factors is consistent not only in the American population but also in other ethnic backgrounds such as African Americans. However, if the researchers wished to generalise the estimated prevalence of hypertension in the Framingham study population to another ethnic group, it may not have been possible.

Usually, descriptive studies have this limitation. The findings of a descriptive research cannot be generalised. This is because the results are specific to the population under investigation. Descriptive studies are primarily concerned with the distribution of characteristics. Therefore, as the population characteristics differ, the findings of different studies may also differ. However, analytical study designs and trials can be generalised, provided the study findings have internal validity. Thus, the generalisability of study findings is based on the study design, study methods and validity.

13.5 SELECTION CRITERIA

In health research, selection criteria of a study population refers to the essential criteria for selecting the study population.

13.5.1 Inclusion and Exclusion Criteria

In health research, the target population is selected by applying a set of clinical and demographic characteristics on a community. Earlier, we discussed that accessible population is selected from the target population by applying certain geographic and temporal characteristics. To select a study sample from the study population, researchers must follow certain selection criteria known as 'inclusion criteria' and 'exclusion criteria'.

Inclusion criteria are the main characteristics of a target population that pertain to the research question. It includes demographic, clinical, geographic and temporal characteristics. On the other hand, exclusion criteria are the characteristics that should not be present in the target population. The presence of exclusion criteria in a study population might interfere with the success of the follow-up efforts or the quality of collected data and the acceptability of the research, or may have ethical concerns. Thus, the characteristics of the target population that the researcher does not want to include in the study are defined as exclusion criteria.

Therefore, while selecting the sample population for a study, one should first define the inclusion criteria. Based on the specific inclusion criteria, an accessible population should be selected. Then, by applying exclusion criteria, unsuitable candidates have to be excluded from the accessible population to derive study samples. For example, the selection criteria for a clinical trial titled, "Does a low dose of Metformin reduce dysmenorrhea in females who have polycystic ovary?" is given below. The research question for this trial was, "What is the lowest dose of Metformin that can help reduce dysmenorrhea in females who have polycystic ovary?" The inclusion criteria are the main characteristics of the population that must be included in the study and are relevant to the research question. In this example, the demographic characteristics of the study population will be females in the reproductive age group of 15–44 years; clinical characteristics would be reproductive females with polycystic ovary and suffering from dysmenorrhea; geographic characteristics can be patients getting treated at a hospital's OPD (study setting) in a specified region; temporal characteristic is the time specified for the study, i.e., from January 1 to December 31 of a specific year. Therefore, these are the inclusion criteria for the study.

The exclusion criteria for the research are:

(i) patients who are already under Metformin therapy for some other diseases like diabetes,

(ii) individuals with hypersensitivity to Metformin,

(iii) individuals with renal dysfunction and

(iv) individuals with contraindication for Metformin.

13.5.2 Clinical Versus Community Study Participants

Researchers must decide the source of the study population—whether it is clinical population or community population. For the previous example, the study participants will be females in the reproductive age group (15–44 years), having clinical characteristics of polycystic ovary and suffering from dysmenorrhea, and getting treated at the OPD of a particular hospital between January 1 and December 31 of a specific year. To obtain internally valid and good quality data, it is preferred that the source of the clinical population is primary healthcare clinics.

However, it is advisable to draw the study population for community-based studies from the community. For example, healthy participants from the community are preferred over hospital population for vaccine efficacy studies. However, in the case of true population-based studies, it is not easy to enumerate house-to-house community population, conduct sampling and include the study participants within a specific period. Moreover, it is expensive to recruit the participants in this manner. But to derive robust public health and clinical decisions for the community, population-based samples would be most appropriate.

13.6 RECRUITMENT

What are the different strategies used for recruiting study participants? What factors should be considered while collecting the study sample?

Feasibility is one of the most important factors that researchers should consider while choosing an accessible population and deciding on sampling methods. Feasibility determines the sampling procedure and how the accessible population is selected from the target population.

In research, the study participants should be representative of the target population, as the study findings depend on the sample population. If the study sample does not represent the intended target population, the results will have errors and will not be internally valid. Hence, while recruiting the study sample, care must be taken to include participants according to the inclusion and exclusion criteria. Another critical aspect of recruitment is adequate sample size. The study must recruit sufficient participants. Otherwise, the result can be biased.

13.7 ACHIEVING A REPRESENTATIVE SAMPLE

How can a researcher achieve a representative sample?

A representative sample can be achieved in the design and implementation phases of the study. In the design phase, the researcher must be cautious in choosing the accessible population from the target population. Additionally, an appropriate sampling method should be used to recruit the study sample from the accessible population. In the implementation phase, the selection criteria should be strictly implemented to prevent selection bias. Following the selection criteria can help achieve a representative study sample. Also, the researcher should closely monitor the study participants throughout the study period. The rate of failure to follow up in case of a longitudinal study and non-response rate must be kept low.

13.8 NON-RESPONSES

While selecting the study population, another critical point to bear in mind is non-responses. In the case of a longitudinal study, failure to follow up can also constitute non-response. Non-responses can influence the internal validity of study findings. When the failure to follow up or non-response rate is high in a study, the sample size will get reduced. This will affect the internal validity of the study. Non-response may also compromise the generalisability of the study. Thus, external validity will be affected.

Now, the question is, how can a researcher address non-responses in a study?

During the design phase, the researcher should determine the adequate sample size, considering the anticipated non-response rate. During the implementation phase, if a participant is unavailable on first contact, repeated attempts should be made to contact the participant, if feasible. Always try to avoid discomfort during the interview and follow-up process. The questionnaire should be simple and understandable to the participants. Usually, the local language of the participants is preferred. In particular, compensating the participants with loss of wage or transportation allowance can help minimise follow-up loss.

Before selecting a study sample from a population, the target population and accessible population must be defined by considering pre-determined inclusion criteria. Then, the study sample must be selected from the accessible population by applying the exclusion criteria. By using an appropriate sampling procedure, the estimated sample size should be selected. Finally, a suitable recruitment strategy must be applied to reduce the non-response rate of the participants.

References and Further Reading

1. Campbell MJ, Swinscow TDV. *Statistics at square one.* 11th ed. United Kingdom: Wiley Blackwell; 2009. Available from: https://www.bmj.com/about-bmj/resources-readers/publications/statistics-square-one/3-populations-and-samples.
2. Weijer C. Selecting subjects for participation in clinical research: one sphere of justice. *J Med Ethics.*1999;25(1):31-6. Available from: http://www.ncbi.nlm.nih.gov/pmc/articles/PMC479165/pdf/jmedeth00002-0035.pdf.
3. Chapter 3 - Research design, research method and population. In: Alannah Allison. p. 84-99. Available from: http://uir.unisa.ac.za/bitstream/handle/10500/1313/04chapter3.pdf.

STUDY PLAN AND PROJECT MANAGEMENT

Sanjay Mehendale

Learning Objectives

At the end of this chapter, readers will be able to:

1. Outline the steps involved in selecting study participants
2. Distinguish between internal validity and external validity
3. Define inclusion and exclusion criteria
4. Recognise and address issues related to non-response

14.1 PRINCIPLES OF PROJECT MANAGEMENT

It is important to spend a lot of time in planning for a project, as only a well-planned study can succeed. If we do not anticipate the eventualities, we might face difficulties while implementing the plan and eventually even in interpreting the study results. This chapter will discuss the systematic process or approach that a researcher can follow to ensure that a research project/study is implemented properly.

In project management, it is crucial to ensure that the defined objectives are adequately met. The specific deliverables that are set at the beginning of the study are intended to be achieved by defining the objectives. The products/deliverables should be completed within the specified timeframe and within the available budget and should meet the set quality standards. The project's result should be able to provide directions for future implications. Any research should help us plan for a better tomorrow. All this can be achieved through effective project management.

Researchers need to follow certain **underlying principles** during the **implementation** of a project to achieve the ultimate **goal successfully**.

The first principle is related to the **process of resource allocation and its management.** The underlying principle here is **time management.** The resources for a project have to be allocated in a timely manner. In a long-term study, the funds need to be disbursed on multiple occasions. Therefore, proper timing is critical to ensure **efficient and practical progress towards achieving the goal.** The second process is **planning and scheduling the activities.** The underlying principle here is **monitoring and supervision, as it helps** to ensure the smooth implementation of the project. Every single detail has to be planned meticulously to achieve the goal of **meeting quality standards.** These principles will guide the smooth conduct of the research.

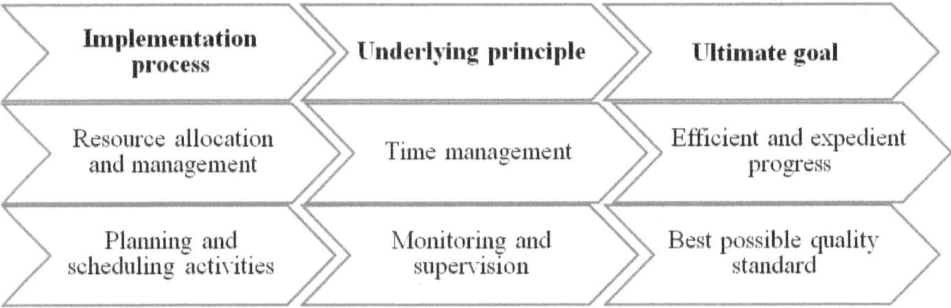

▲ **Figure 14.1:** Principles of project management

14.2 NON-PRODUCTIVE AD HOC APPROACH

Ad hoc decisions taken while conducting a research are often non-productive. At the beginning of a study, there can be a lot of uncertainty in the minds of researchers such as, "I want to conduct a study, but I am not clear about the objectives" or "I have prepared a questionnaire, but I am not clear about the exact information I need" or "I will collect the data, but I am not clear how I should use that".

Such confusions arise because of lack of clarity on the research topic. The result of such analyses can be disastrous. It will lead to the generation of data that is difficult to analyse. The analysed data can then become difficult to interpret, and even when interpretations are made, they may not be of use to the programme or policymaking. Hence, an ad hoc approach taken without proper planning is unlikely to succeed.

14.3 ANALYSIS PLAN

Any research process typically starts with identifying the need for the research, then goes through various stages such as correctly spelling out the research question, formulating the study objectives, planning the analysis, preparing data collection instruments, collecting data, analysing data, drawing appropriate conclusions, developing specific recommendations and involving the stakeholders from the programme.

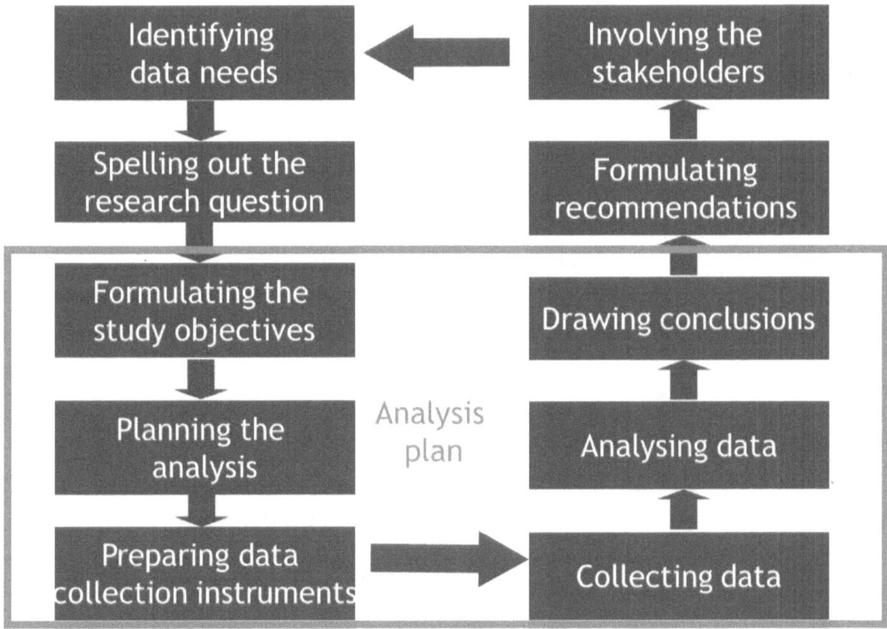

▲ **Figure 14.2:** Steps for conducting a research

While conducting a research, we have to assess whether the needs of our research, which were identified initially, are fulfilled or not. Identifying data needs and spelling out the research question comprise the pre-planning phase. These activities are done much before the study is conceptualised. Formulating the objectives, analysing the data and drawing conclusions form part of the planning and implementation phase. Then comes disseminating the findings to the concerned stakeholders to aid in proper programmatic absorption or policymaking.

14.4 ROADMAP TO PLANNING AND MANAGING A STUDY

The roadmap to planning and managing a study involves the following steps:

1. Formulate appropriate objectives for the study.
2. Choose the right design to determine critical indicators.
3. Decide on a suitable study design for the research question.
4. Estimate the sample size before the investigation.
5. Identify the parameters needed for the key indicators of the study.
6. Prepare an outline for analysis.

Researchers must keep in mind that studies conducted on small samples may not be generalisable.

14.5 FRAMING STUDY OBJECTIVES

There are a few basic principles for framing study objectives. The fewer the objectives, the better it is. Studies that have a long list of objectives tend to get very complex. As the data collection tools increase, there may be variations in collecting the data, which can cause the objectives stated in the protocol to remain unfulfilled. Thus, it is prudent to stop with a few objectives, depending on the feasibility.

Objectives can be categorised as primary objectives and secondary objectives. The primary objective is crucial as it helps to decide the sample size for the study. Often, sample size is calculated based on the condition that we should at least be able to achieve the primary objective. Secondary objectives are the analysable issues and the additional information that we obtain during a research.

Objectives should be clearly phrased. They can be of two types: exploratory and confirmatory. The exploratory type is aimed at testing a hypothesis. For example, "to determine whether a contaminated well caused an outbreak of a disease". The confirmatory type is aimed at measuring a quantity. For example, "to estimate the prevalence of diabetes in a community". Appropriate verbs should be used while defining the objectives.

14.6 CHOICE OF STUDY DESIGN

Different study designs are adopted to answer different types of research questions—usually, descriptive objectives are used for exploring **acute conditions**. For example, consider the following objective: "To estimate the number of children with pneumonia or diarrhoea and its aetiology in a community". The appropriate study design for this objective would be a **cohort study or a surveillance study**, which may include hospital-based or community-based surveillance. The measure of disease frequency used in a cohort study is **incidence.**

Chronic conditions occur for a long time, and individuals are either treated or not treated. The measure of disease frequency used in such kinds of studies is **prevalence**. The appropriate study design for such studies is **cross-sectional study**.

Some epidemiological studies also involve **comparing two groups**. For example, comparing (i) individuals exposed to a particular condition with (ii) individuals not exposed to the particular condition; or comparing (i) individuals suffering from a particular disease with (ii) individuals not suffering from the particular disease. When the direction of enquiry is from the variable or the exposure to the outcome, we call it a **cohort study. A cohort study** is a **prospective** assessment. On the other hand, when the direction of enquiry is from outcome to exposure, it is a **retrospective** assessment. In this case, the outcome or the disease of interest has already occurred. The study design to be used here is a **case-control study**.

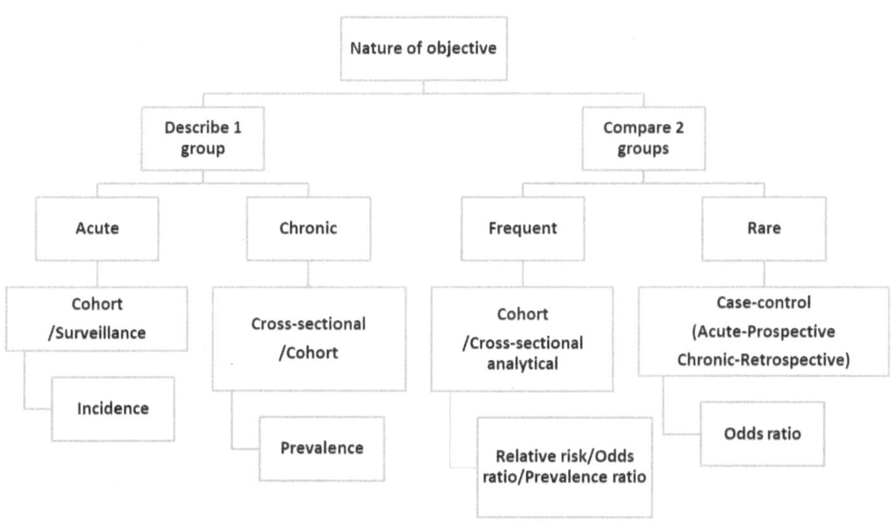

▲ **Figure 14.3:** Choice of study design and measures of disease frequency

A **cohort study** should be undertaken only when the outcome is likely to **occur frequently**. If the outcome of interest occurs over a long period of time, the study will go on for that long, and the adequate number of outcomes may not be achieved. However, for **frequently occurring** outcomes, the duration from exposure to the outcome is likely to be minimal. In such instances, a **cohort study** is a good approach, or alternatively a **cross-sectional analytical study** can be undertaken.

In case of **rare exposures** and when the duration between exposure and outcome is likely to be very long, a **case-control approach** is recommended. The measures to be used to determine the magnitude of association are odds ratio and relative risk ratio for case-control and cohort studies respectively. Relative risk is a better indicator of the magnitude of association than odds ratio.

14.7 INFORMATION REQUIRED FOR CALCULATING INDICATORS

During the planning phase, due emphasis has to be given to collecting the information required for framing the indicators for the study. The indicators can be rates, ratios, proportions or quantitative variables.

Researchers need to plan to identify and collect the information related to the numerators and denominators required to determine the indicators. Besides, the elements required to calculate indicators such as outcome variables and covariates like potential risk factors and confounders should also be listed.

14.8 PRINCIPLES TO BE FOLLOWED WHILE COLLECTING THE INFORMATION ELEMENTS

Researchers should include the variables that will best reflect the information required after reviewing the available evidence through a literature search. The review, when performed rigorously, will provide the researcher with proof of which variables or covariates are essential for the study. Researchers must collect only those variables that will be used for analysis.

It is important to use validated or standardised methods and criteria that are replicable elsewhere too. Standardised case definitions have to be adopted in the research. For example, a researcher wants to estimate the prevalence of pneumonia among children under the age of five in a community. Here, the researcher should come up with a clear operational definition of what constitutes pneumonia. Another researcher wishes to evaluate the association between smoking and cardiovascular disease among women of reproductive age in a community. Here, smoking is the exposure variable. The researcher has to provide an operational definition of how to classify a person as a smoker—

whether it is based on ever smoked history as "yes or no", or based on the frequency of smoking or the number of cigarettes smoked per day.

Similarly, in research involving laboratory parameters, standard criteria and normal ranges should be decided based on available evidence. For example, if a researcher conducts a study on anaemia, the operational definition or normative values of what constitutes anaemia and what does not have to be clearly spelt out with respect to age and gender.

Researchers should decide on the most reliable and accurate way of collecting the required information. The information can be collected through observation, interviews using a questionnaire or laboratory assays.

14.9 OUTCOME MEASUREMENT

The table below (Table 14.1) provides a summary of the outcomes, information elements required and the method of data collection for each element, for a study on iodine deficiency disorder among adults in India.

▼ **Table 14.1:** Outcomes, information elements and methods of data collection for a study on iodine deficiency disorder among adults in India

Outcome	Information element	Data collection method
Chronic iodine deficiency	Goitre	Physical examination
Current exposure to iodine	Iodine excretion in urine	Laboratory test
Access to iodized salt	Testing household salt for iodine	Field spot test

The most appropriate and feasible method of data collection should be chosen depending on the objective, exposure and outcome variables. Besides the direction, there may also be other potential risk factors or confounders that should be collected to get an accurate picture of why a particular outcome occurs. These are called covariates. In the above example, there can be **risk factors** like **income**, **community** (e.g. minorities), education, **social and cultural** practices, and **dietary patterns** that may profoundly influence the outcome. Therefore, they should be included in the analysis and the interpretation of results.

Similarly, the risk of contracting a disease might vary with **age**, **gender** and place of **residence**. These are **confounding factors** as they affect both the exposure and the outcome variable. It is crucial to include and collect information on all known confounders in the questionnaire. The results need to be analysed after adjusting for confounders.

14.10 ADVANTAGES OF ANALYSIS PLAN

Preparing an analysis plan helps researchers focus on the study objectives. They can also prepare dummy tables at the beginning of the study to make each objective clear. An analysis plan helps to avoid unnecessary comparison of information that is not important for the study. It ensures that only data that is required for the analysis is collected. It saves time by facilitating speedy publication, dissemination of findings and early policy feedback. Thence, a detailed analytical plan has to be prepared.

14.11 SAMPLE SIZE

The sample size must be estimated depending on the outcome assessment based on measurement or testing. The method of sample size calculation will differ based on the study design: whether it is a cohort study, case-control study or cross-sectional study and whether it is a descriptive study or an analytical study. Therefore, it is essential to involve a statistician right from the time of estimating the sample size for the study until the analysis stage.

14.12 REASONS FOR STUDY FAILURES

The following are a few reasons why a study could become a failure:

- Poorly defined research questions and unclear objectives that can lead to disastrous results
- Unrealistic timelines that may be too short or too long
- Incompetent staff who lack direction, motivation and training
- Inadequate monitoring
- Failure to respond to contingent situations
- Carrying out mid-course corrections that can result in a catastrophe

14.13 ATTENTION POINTS IN STUDY / PROJECT MANAGEMENT

There are several factors that aid the successful completion of a study. Human resource management is a critical aspect of project management. The study staff should be carefully chosen and appropriately trained. Effective communication is a crucial factor for the effective implementation of a project. The project manager should encourage conflict-free team dynamics and rapport among the project staff to ensure effective communication. Time management is the responsibility of the leader. An effective leader must provide the appropriate scheduling of various activities on time.

Financial management is the next important thing as the research project may progress well with the initial funding but may slow down due to delays in the disbursement of subsequent instalments. Therefore, researchers must give due importance to financial management to ensure smooth execution of the project. The following are some examples of the financial aspects that need to be taken care of:

- A clear financial plan for the project
- The number of instalments
- The amount of funds that has to be released in each instalment
- Timeline for release of funds and alternative strategies in case of any delays

Next, the researcher should ensure that quality management for data collection, clinical and laboratory procedures, data management and a plan for supervisory visits are in place. Quality management is crucial for the successful completion of projects. Emphasis should be given to timely data management. If there are any issues in data collection, a regular and timely assessment will help rectify the errors mid-course rather than at the end of the study when rectification may not be possible. Teamwork and coordination among the project staff and adequate monitoring of the progress and targets achieved are other factors that can help ensure the successful completion of a study. The mechanism used to monitor the study can be either internal or external. As mentioned earlier, each of the factors should be considered individually and collectively during the planning, implementation and completion of the project.

References and Further Reading

1. United Nations Children's Fund, United Nations Development Programme, World Bank,WHO Special Programme for Research and Training in Tropical Disease. Effective project planning and evaluation in biomedical research: a step by step guide: participants. Geneva: World Health Organization; 2005. https://apps.who.int/iris/bitstream/handle/10665/69237/TDR_RCS_PPE_05.2_eng.pdf?sequence=2

CHAPTER 15

DESIGNING DATA COLLECTION TOOLS

Tarun Bhatnagar

Learning Objectives

At the end of this chapter, readers will be able to:

1. Explain the various types of data collection tools
2. Describe the components of a data collection tool
3. Define the procedure for constructing a data collection tool
4. Outline the design of a data collection tool

In this chapter, readers will be given an overview of how to design data collection tools or instruments that are used to collect data in health research.

15.1 INFORMATION COLLECTED USING DATA COLLECTION TOOLS

In health research, researchers collect information in three areas—facts, knowledge and judgment—as shown in Figure 15.1. Facts include the study participants' characteristics, the environment they live in and their behaviours or practices. In the knowledge section, researchers may want to know about the participants' knowledge of risk factors for acquiring a disease or healthy lifestyles to prevent infections. In the judgement section, they may wish to collect information on the participants' judgment, such as their opinions and attitudes. For example, "What are the opinions of the research participants on the quality of health services provided at primary health centres?" Another example is, "What are the respondents' attitudes towards adherence to anti-hypertensive medication, open-air defaecation or seat belt usage?"

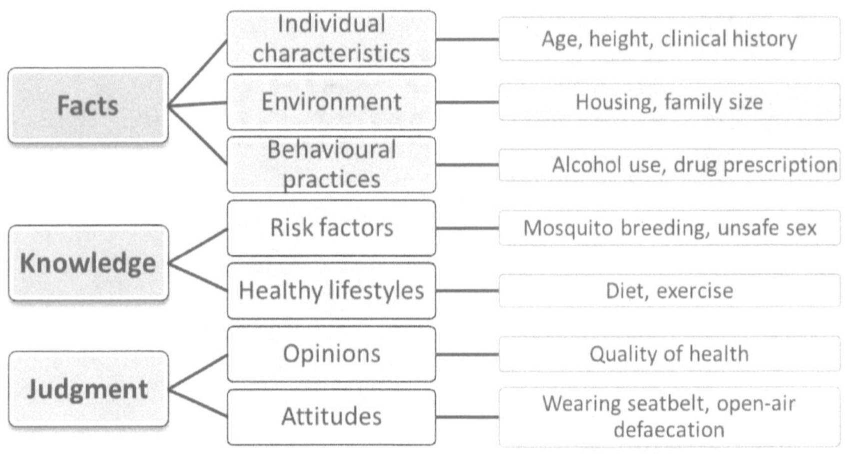

▲ **Figure 15.1:** Information commonly collected using data collection tools

15.2 TOOLS USED TO COLLECT DATA

Researchers use a variety of tools to collect data, depending on the kind of data they wish to collect. Data collection tools are categorised as: abstraction form, structured observation guide and questionnaire. Researchers use an abstraction form to collect data by reviewing participant records, which can be their records/forms. One can look at the clinical records of individuals to obtain information on their disease condition, signs and symptoms, and treatment given. Besides individual and aggregate information, one can also gather data from existing disease surveillance records. In addition, data can be collected from existing registers. The information from all these sources can be gathered in a data abstraction form.

A structured observation guide is another data collection tool that is used to document specific processes. For example, is a particular procedure happening or not? If so, how is it happening? Is it happening on time or not? Are the objectives of the study met? To collect such information, researchers may use a checklist of items that could be either textual or figurative.

The third and most commonly used tool for data collection is a **questionnaire** that data collectors use to interact with the participants in person and gather information. Questionnaires are of two types: **interviewer-administered** and **self-administered**. In the former, the data collector interviews the respondents using a questionnaire, either **face-to-face or** over **telephone or** using **computer-assisted technologies**. Later, the data collector hands out the questionnaire to the participants, who fill in the required information after reading through the questions. Self-administered questionnaires can either be **paper-based** or **computer-assisted. Computer-assisted** questionnaires allow respondents to feed their information directly into a computer database. Participant literacy is a prerequisite for self-administered questionnaires.

15.3 KEY ELEMENTS OF DATA COLLECTION TOOLS

Irrespective of the type of data collection tool, valid responses from participants are a must. The responses should be relevant and helpful to meet the research requirements. The following factors should be kept in mind while designing a data collection tool:

- Clarity of **words**
- **Balance** between phrases and sentences
- **Length of sentences** and **comprehensiveness of responses**

If there are categories for participant responses, researchers can design **constraints** regarding what information can or cannot be collected using the designed data collection tool. In addition, the **utility of the data collection tool**, the **utility of the instructions** and the **precise order** in which the questions are asked are crucial factors that determine how participants answer the questions. Above all, the **context** in which the questions are framed and the tools used have to be borne in mind.

15.4 COMPONENTS OF A DATA COLLECTION TOOL

A data collection tool generally has four components: an introduction at the beginning and a conclusion at the end, identifiers, instructions for data collectors and the instrument's body, which contains the questions.

The **introduction** part introduces the study, states the objectives, explains the study's purpose and procedure for data collection, and gets informed consent from the participants. The **concluding statement** is presented at the end of the questionnaire, thanking the study participants for their time and effort in answering the questions.

Every data collection tool will have **identifiers** such as the name and address of the participant, using which one can identify the participant. In conformance to the principles of ethics and confidentiality, researchers should collect identifier information in a separate sheet of paper that can be referred to later on, if required. Researchers can also maintain confidentiality by assigning coded identification numbers to the participants. These identification numbers could be a composite code of text and numbers denoting, for example, the state, district, village and household. If there are more than one participant from each household, individual numbers can be assigned for each participant. The composite code so derived would be unique for each participant. Such a code will serve the promise of privacy protection and confidentiality, and no one other than the investigator will know the basic identifying information of the participants.

The next component is **instructions for data collectors**. This can be general, such as **prompts**. For example: "do not read out all the responses" or "tick only the one response that the study participant mentions". The researcher can also give instructions on **skip patterns** when subsequent questions may not be relevant to the participant. For example: "If the participant is a non-smoker, then skip questions 2–6 and go to question number 7". This means that questions 2–6 are relevant only if the participant is a smoker. It is advisable to use **a different font style** to clearly distinguish between the actual questions and instructions for the data collector.

The last component is the **body of the instrument**, which contains the question items. These question items could be of various types: **open questions, closed-ended questions** or **semi-open questions.**

15.5 OPEN QUESTIONS

As the name indicates, open questions will not provide any suggestions regarding the answer; the respondents will have to generate their own responses for such questions. Here, the participants will have complete freedom to answer the questions as they please. There will be no categories of answers to constrain them. This helps stimulate the memory of the participants, thereby facilitating a better response. Besides, it is also helpful at the hypothesis generation stage when researchers may be unsure about the appropriate answer. However, the downside of this type of questions is that they can generate a lot of varied responses from the study participants, which may pose difficulties in coding and analysis. Researchers may get a long list of answers that might be difficult to categorise. At times, open responses may be unfocused or incomplete, posing a challenge during analysis.

15.6 OPEN QUESTIONS WITH CLOSED-ENDED ANSWERS

To overcome the problem of incomplete responses, researchers can continue to have open questions but with closed-ended answers. In this type of questions, categories of answers will be given for the questions. However, the data collector will not suggest a response from these categories. As and when the participant provides the answers, the interviewer will spontaneously make a note under the corresponding categories. Although such questions are expressed as open questions, they are considered as closed-ended questions.

Example: What practices may increase your risk of getting a heart attack? (DO NOT propose any option for the answer)

1. Lack of exercise (Yes/No)
2. Smoking (Yes/No)
3. Poor dietary practices (Yes/No)
4. Overeating salt (Yes/No)

15.7 CLOSED-ENDED QUESTIONS

Closed-ended questions are questions that have a set category of answers that are acceptable to the researcher. They can be dichotomous or have multiple options. Examples of dichotomous options are yes/no, male/female, etc.

For example: "Did you eat at restaurant X between 1st and 28th February? Yes/No

"Have you ever consumed tobacco products? Yes/No

Closed-ended questions help respondents take a clear position. Such questions are instrumental in getting the participants to focus on key information, especially for critical issues. However, they may oversimplify the response for certain issues where dichotomous answers may yield inadequate information.

A closed-ended question with multiple options, as the name indicates, can have more than one response. For this type of questions, the researcher can ask the questions and then ask the participants to choose one or more answers from the options provided for the particular question.

Examples:
"Where do you go to seek treatment for fever?" (Multiple answers are permitted)

1. Government hospital
2. Private clinic
3. Pharmacist
4. Traditional healer

"Do you wear a helmet while riding a bike? (Select only one answer)

1. Always
2. Sometimes
3. Never

While designing a questionnaire, researchers have to provide clear instructions for the data collector as to whether only one or more than one answer is acceptable. Researchers have to be mindful of the possibility of multiple probable options while designing questionnaires to prevent confusion.

There are also closed-ended questions that can have quantitative answers. For such questions, respondents have to provide a number, such as age. For example: "How many times did you visit the clinic in the last 12 months?" This question requires the participant to respond with a continuous variable that can be analysed or categorised later at the time of analysis.

Here is another example: "How would you rate your pain level on a scale of 1–10?" (where 1 and 10 indicate the minimum and maximum pain levels, respectively). The variable here is qualitative with ten options and requires validation. A participant with a score of six may not be a double three on the scale. Hence, the quantified answers may be limited in how they can be handled as continuous variables. Sometimes, the number can itself be challenging to interpret. All these points have to be taken into consideration while framing questions.

15.8 SEMI-OPEN QUESTIONS

Semi-open questions have several response options. Participants can choose their answer from the options suggested or provide their own response in the open option provided. The most common open option in data collection tools and questionnaires is 'others'.

For example: "Did your child have complications following measles?

1. None
2. Pneumonia
3. Diarrhoea
4. Eye problems
5. Others, specify____________

Here, the specific complications given may be the common ones seen. Besides these, there may be other uncommon complications, which the respondent can provide in the "Others" field. This type of questions permit the capturing of any unplanned answers. However, if the questionnaire contains many such questions, the collected data might become difficult to analyse.

15.9 FORMULATING QUESTIONS

Researchers must follow certain principles while formulating questions for a questionnaire. The questions should be **short and precise**. For example, if a researcher wants to know the age of the study participant, merely writing 'age' alone in the questionnaire is not a good idea. Always use complete phrases, like "What is your age?", to **avoid ambiguities**. It is better to **use simple words** rather than complicated or academic ones. Use everyday language for framing questions as the respondents are often laypeople. It is ideal to **avoid negatives and double negatives**. For example, consider the following question: "Do you sometimes care for patients **without** washing hands?" There is a negative connotation here. Also, there are two parts to this question—one is 'caring for patients' and the other is 'without washing hands'. A better way to phrase this question would be to ask it directly and with a positive note—"Do you systematically wash your hands before caring for each patient?" This question is unambiguous and also avoids negatives.

Next, each question should **focus on one idea** only. For example, consider the following question: "Did you refuse treatment because you feared side effects?" There are actually two ideas in this question—one asks if the respondent had refused treatment, and the other asks why the respondent refused treatment. If the respondent had not refused treatment, then they would not be able to answer the question. Therefore, it is better to split such questions into two. The first part can be reframed as: "Did you refuse treatment?", and if the answer to the above question is 'Yes', the follow-up question could be, "Was this because you feared side effects?" The questions are now straightforward and easy to comprehend.

The questions should be **specific**. For example, a researcher wants to know the respondents' awareness about how HIV is transmitted and puts forth the question: "Are you aware of the modes of HIV transmission?" This is an open-ended question that permits respondents to answer whatever they want. Suppose the researcher wants to narrow down to specifics as to whether HIV is transmitted through heterosexual or homosexual route, blood transfusion, drug use, etc. In that case, it is better to rephrase the question as: "Which of the following practices could expose you to HIV?" Then the answer options could be given to choose from. There is a better chance of getting appropriate answers for the rephrased question.

It is better to **use a neutral tone** and **avoid judgmental tones** since they may influence the response of the study participants. A data collector should remain non-judgmental and record participant responses without any prejudice. For example, a researcher wants to know about the sexual practices of individuals, and so asks the question: "Have you been promiscuous in the last six months?" The word 'promiscuous' has a negative connotation here. It can be more neutral, direct and specific, such as, "How many sexual partners have you had in the last six months?"

15.10 SORTING THE ORDER OF QUESTIONS

The questions listed in a questionnaire should have a conversational flow. There should be a smooth flow of questions, from one to the next. The following are some general principles to keep in mind while sorting questions. Ask simple questions first and keep the complicated questions for the later part. Ask generic questions such as socio-demographic characteristics first and then move on to specific questions relevant to the study. Ask more casual questions in the beginning, to build a rapport with the respondent. Then continue with the factual questions and questions on intimate or sensitive issues. Questions about attitudes and opinions can be asked later on in the interview. Group together all questions that are related to the same topic of enquiry. If questions related to a single topic are spread across different parts of the questionnaire, it can confuse the respondent. Ask identification questions such as name, age, gender and address either at the beginning or at the end.

If the researcher wants to collect information about a sequence of events, then the questions should be asked in the chronological order of how things would have happened in real-time. This approach will help respondents recall the incident in a better and more logical way. If the questionnaire is complex with many questions, give a break in the middle. Complex questions can follow a few simple questions. Sometimes, researchers may ask the same kind of question in different ways if the subject matter is essential for the study. This can help the researcher understand and validate the participant's response.

15.11 LAYING OUT THE DATA COLLECTION TOOL

Once the order of the questions is sorted, the focus should shift to the layout of the questions in the questionnaire. The structure of the questionnaire can influence how participants respond. Different subjects covered in the questionnaire should be split into different sections, with a line between sections for demarcation. Adequate space must be provided between the questions to make them easily readable. The font size should be large enough to facilitate easy reading. A font size of 11 or 12 would be ideal. Questions should not be split across pages. If a question is split across two pages, the data collector will have to turn the page while reading the question. This can make it difficult for the data collector to read the question and convey its meaning to the participant. Therefore, questions should not be split across pages. Questions should be aligned neatly. It is good to align questions on the left-hand side and answers and codes on the right-hand side. This would help distinguish between the two columns and make it visually appealing.

Number the questions in ascending order, starting from 1, 2, etc. All responses should be coded and entered into the software of choice for analysis. Therefore, it is advisable to have a standardised coding system built into the questionnaire itself.

Let us now look at a few examples for coding of responses. In case of a dichotomous response such as 'Yes/ No', the researcher can apply a code of 1 for 'Yes' and 0 for 'No'. Every question/response with 'Yes/No' options can be coded as 1 and 0, respectively. Let's say a researcher has 'Male/Female' as the response for gender. 'Male' can be coded as 1 and 'Female' can be coded as 2.

Another simple way of coding is auto-coding. For example, if there are four response options, they will be numbered as 1, 2, 3 and 4. If the second option is selected, number 2 will be recorded as the code for this question.

The layout of the questionnaire has to be neat and presentable. The points discussed so far will help make the questionnaire handy for the data collector, the data entry operator and the statistician who will analyse the data at a later stage.

15.12 FINALISING THE DATA COLLECTION TOOL

While finalising the data collection tool, the researcher has to check whether the questions in the tool are relevant to the study. Essentially, the researcher needs to be a slave of the objectives and the pre-planned analysis of the survey. Only questions that are relevant to the study objectives should be retained in the questionnaire. All other unnecessary questions should be removed. Researchers should also check for any missing queries and add them. The questionnaire should be reviewed before the initiation of data collection. Colleagues called peer reviewers or experts in the field can review the tool. The statistician should also review the coding used in the tool. This would be helpful for analysis at a later stage. The field workers and data entry operators engaged in the study should also review the data collection tool. The questionnaire can also be given to key informants to check whether the flow of questions is appropriate, whether the questions make sense, and to look for any ambiguities or difficulties in comprehension.

The data collection tool, the questionnaire or the data abstraction form has to be in the language in which the researcher will interview the study participants. The questionnaire should use a language that is convenient for the participants to understand.

Since English is the common official language, researchers may initially frame the questionnaire in English. However, it has to be translated into the local language and re-translated back into English to ensure that the translated version in the local language makes the same sense as the initial questions in English.

15.13 PILOT TESTING THE DATA COLLECTION TOOL

Before implementing a study, it is essential to pilot test the data collection tool. The researcher needs to check whether the study instrument is precise and the questions are understandable and acceptable to the study participants. The flow and the skip patterns in the tool should also be checked. This will help in ensuring that the coding works as expected and give a sense of the time that would be taken by the participants to answer the questionnaire. Pilot testing can be done by administering the questionnaire to a few volunteers who are similar to the study population. However, these individuals on whom pilot testing was done should not be included later on in the main study.

15.14 DESIGNING HEALTH RESEARCH TOOLS

While designing health research tools, researchers have to decide how to measure the concepts and relate them to the study design and objectives. Then, they have to match the scale for the chosen measures to plan the analysis. The scales, questions, questionnaires and data collection tools should be reliable and valid for the study population. The researcher should choose the most appropriate data collection method, whether it is a data abstraction form, a structured observation guide or a questionnaire, along with the type of questions to be used in the data collection instrument. Everything should be planned in the data collection tool keeping the study participants in mind, such as the language of the questionnaire, method of measuring the concepts and the best way of asking the actual questions.

A study questionnaire can make or break a study. Once researchers collect the data, they may not have the opportunity to return to the participants. Therefore, it is essential to collect valid and reliable data at the time of data collection. Also, it is critical to ensure that the data collection instruments are valid and appropriate for the study.

References and Further Reading

1. Bellary S, Krishnankutty B, Latha MS. Basics of case report form designing in clinical research. PerspectClin Res 2014;5(4):159-66. http://www.ncbi.nlm.nih.gov/pmc/articles/PMC4170533/
2. Global Health Trials.Downloadable templates and tools for clinical research. https://globalhealthtrials.tghn.org/articles/downloadable-templates-and-tools-clinical-research/

CHAPTER 16 PRINCIPLES OF DATA COLLECTION

Prabhdeep Kaur

Learning Objectives

At the end of this chapter, readers will be able to:

1. Describe the essential steps in data collection
2. Identify the approaches to ensure data quality during data collection

The previous chapter discussed different data collection tools, study plans and project management. In this chapter, we will talk about the principles of data collection. Data collection is one of the essential components of a research study because this step will determine the quality of data that you will gather in your research.

16.1 PRINCIPLES OF DATA QUALITY

There are two main principles of data quality—**reliability and accuracy**.

Reliability and Accuracy

Reliability or repeatability means that if different investigators repeat the same study or the exact measurements, they should get similar results. Reliability also refers to the stability and consistency of the information collected.

Reliability alone does not ensure that the gathered data is of good quality; the data has to be accurate. Accuracy refers to the extent to which a measurement is correctly done. Sometimes, the collected data could be both reliable and accurate, or both the attributes may not be present simultaneously.

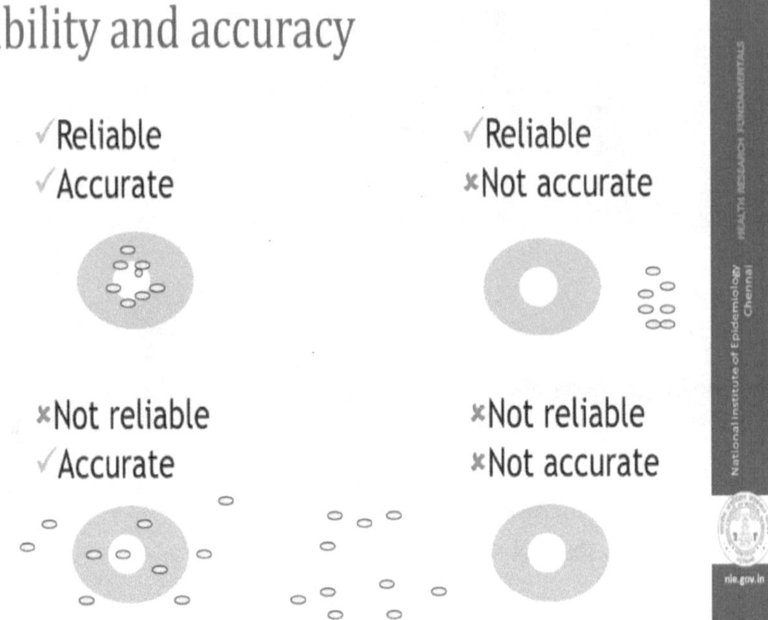

▲ **Figure 16.1:** Reliability and accuracy of data

As shown in Figure 16.1, your study can give you a reliable and accurate result, which means your data offer the precise measurement you want. In such a scenario, if you repeat the measure, it will approximately provide the same result each time. However, this is an ideal case scenario. In a worst-case scenario, your measurement could be both inaccurate and unreliable. There can be other possibilities as well, where your measurement is reliable but inaccurate or accurate but not reliable. Therefore, a good quality research study must ensure that the data collected in the study are accurate and reliable.

16.2 SIX STEPS IN DATA COLLECTION

There are six broad steps that have to be followed during data collection.

1. Draft a question-by-question guide
2. Train the staff members
3. Initiate data collection and pilot testing
4. Conduct periodic reviews of collected data to ensure quality and completeness

5. Debrief to troubleshoot difficulties
6. Validate the study results

Now, we will discuss each of these steps in detail.

16.2.1 Drafting the Question-By-Question Guide

Question-by-question guide is a short, simple document that will guide field workers and research staff during data collection.

Why is the question-by-question guide essential for data collection? It is very important because there must be uniformity in interviewing participants. Different data collectors may understand the same question differently. Each of your staff members may have their own interpretations of how a particular question needs to be asked and how it needs to be explained to the respondent. The question-by-question guide ensures that all investigators ask the questions in a uniform manner and have a similar understanding of the questions. In a question-by-question guide, the researcher should briefly explain how the data collectors should ask each of the questions. The guide should also explain the possible responses to the questions. For open-ended questions or qualitative interviews, necessary probes should be included in the question-by-question guide. The guide should also direct the data collector on where to skip and where to emphasise. In essence, the guide should serve as a roadmap for data collection. So, whenever there is a doubt or a lack of consistency among data collectors and researchers, they can review the question-by-question guide to ensure consistent data collection.

Often, during data collection, data collectors or researchers may encounter different difficulties in the field, for which modifications may need to be made in the data collection tool. The researcher must record all these changes in the question-by-question guide.

For example, suppose, in a questionnaire, one question is, "what type of house does the participant live in?" The response to this question could be 'kaccha', 'pucca' or 'semi pucca'. However, everybody may not understand these terms.

Therefore, the question-by-question guide must provide guidance in the following manner: Observe the participant's house.

- If the house is made of mud, thatch or other low-quality materials, mark it as a kaccha house;
- If the house is made of partly low-quality and partly high-quality materials, mark it as a semi-pucca house;
- If the house is made with bricks or high-quality materials throughout, including the floor, roof and exterior walls, mark it as a pucca house.

In this manner, if the meaning of 'kaccha', 'pucca' and 'semi pucca' house is explained in the question-by-question guide, it will be easy for the data collectors and researchers to identify the type of house in the field.

Similarly, suppose you are asking a question regarding household income. There may be multiple earning members in a family. In this case, the researcher should direct the data collectors to first inquire about the number of earning members in the family, then move on to what the monthly income of each member is, and finally calculate the family's total monthly income by adding all the amounts.

16.2.2 Training the Staff Members

Once the question-by-question guide is prepared, the researcher can move on to data collection. However, before starting the data collection, it is essential to ensure that the data collectors are adequately trained to maintain excellent quality of the data. The first step in this process is to recruit appropriate candidates as data collectors. The researcher should recruit suitable data collectors or interviewers for data collection, bearing in mind the requirements of the study. Suppose a researcher wants to conduct a clinical research, then the data collectors must know how to ask clinical questions and how to use clinical terms when interacting with the patients. In the case of a field-based study, the researchers need to ensure that the data collectors are familiar with the local language and know how to interact culturally with the people at the community level.

After recruiting suitable personnel for the study, the researcher has to arrange a training session for them. In this training, the researcher should introduce the purpose and objectives of the study, the data collection tools, operational definitions and the type of data. For example, if your research study is on hypertension, you will have to identify hypertensive people by measuring the participants' blood pressure. You also have to collect various demographic and other data through interviews. Therefore, your study would consist of different components like a questionnaire, followed by measurements.

In this case, you should familiarise your data collectors with various data collection tools and techniques. You should share the question-by-question guide with them, allow them to read each question and ask for their interpretation of the questions. Following this, you should briefly describe to them the steps to be followed in the field and explain how to work with the questionnaire. You could also conduct role-plays by assigning one person as the interviewer and another as a respondent and getting them to enact a mock interview during the training. In this way, you could guide the data collection team to ensure uniform data quality.

16.2.3 Data Collection and Pilot Testing

After training the data collection team, the researcher can initiate data collection. However, training alone does not confirm that the data collection team will be able to perform in a similar way as they did during the training because the actual world situation may be very different when compared to the training platform. Some of the team members may be new to the situation. For example, a data collector may be trained in clinical research but might have never worked in a clinical setting, or a field data collector may be a graduate in social work but might have never worked in a community setting. Pilot testing is an essential step in research study that can help solve this issue.

Pilot testing is a small-scale research study that helps test data collection instruments and techniques before applying them to the primary research project. In pilot testing, data collectors conduct interviews in a setting that is almost similar to the study setting/area. Through piloting, problems in the study instrument and potential areas of difficulties in implementing the research can be identified and solved before initiating the main investigation.

Thus, pilot testing helps the researcher explain and clarify the doubts of data collectors and solve the deficiencies in the process of implementing a research. Before initiating data collection, the researcher must appoint a supervisor who will monitor the data collectors consistently and verify the questionnaires every day in the group. Daily checking of forms is necessary because once the interviewers have left the study area/setting, errors in the forms cannot be corrected.

Moreover, once data collection starts, different problems may arise. The researcher must be available to address these problems. This could be done over the phone or through messages too. Once the data collection has begun, the principal investigator or lead researcher should visit a few on-site study areas to ensure that the data collection is being done as per protocol. This will help ensure the quality of the filled-up questionnaires. The researcher should also keep in mind the time available to complete these questionnaires. However, the pressure on the data collectors to complete the study on time should not compromise the quality of information being gathered.

16.2.4 Reviewing Collected Data for Quality and Completeness

During data collection, researchers may want to review the data collection process to ensure that the collected data is complete and of good quality. There are two ways to do this. The first way is to review the collected data at the data collection site itself. At the end of each day, the supervisor can collect all the forms from the team members and check them on that day itself. The second way is to arrange for the forms to be sent to the researcher, and then go through them.

Checks to be conducted: Now, what kind of checks can researchers do once they get the filled-in forms?

The first and foremost crucial check is to ensure that the forms are complete. When there are many questions in the questionnaire, some of them may be left blank. Therefore, the researcher must ensure the completeness of the data. The second check is readability. The way the questions are marked or clinical symptoms or narratives are described must be readable to others. The third check is consistency. Do the answers make sense? Does the researcher feel that this is how the participants would have answered? Or do the answers indicate that the respondents did not understand the questions?

16.2.5 Debriefing to Troubleshoot Difficulties

Periodic reviews are essential for any study, whether it is a clinical study or a field study.

Supervisors need to conduct periodic review meetings, once a week/month, depending on the duration of the study, whether on-site or off-site. These meetings will help clarify any queries that data collectors have, about the questionnaires. Sometimes, it may be necessary to change the sequencing of questions or responses during data collection. In such cases, the supervisors must ensure that these changes are well-documented and added to the question-by-question guide.

16.2.6 Validation of Study Results

The last important step in data collection is data validation.

A small subsample (could be as small as even 5 per cent) of the study participants should be selected, and an independent second interview must be conducted to validate the collected data. This process will help ensure that the collected data are valid. By comparing the results of the second interview with that of the first interview, the researcher can determine if there are any discrepancies or significant errors in the data collection. This process could also help identify whether a data collector might have been committing specific mistakes that have been repeated across the team. Accordingly, the researcher can discuss the issue with the individual team member or the whole study team.

Before beginning data collection, researchers must understand data quality concepts. Good training of data collectors both in the classroom and on-site in a similar study setting is essential for a good research study. Moreover, supportive supervision and teamwork are key to quality data collection.

References and Further Reading

1. Boynton PM. Administering, analysing, and reporting your questionnaire. *BMJ*. 2004; 328:1372-5.
2. Phillips-Salimi CR, Donovan Stickler MA, Stegenga K, Lee M, Haase JE. Principles and strategies for monitoring data collection integrity in a multi-site randomized clinical trial of a behavioral intervention. *Res Nurs Health*. 2011;34(4):362-71.

DATA MANAGEMENT

P. Manickam

Learning Objectives

At the end of this chapter, readers will be able to:

1. Outline the basic structure of a database
2. Identify issues related to data storage
3. Recognise the elements of data entry
4. Distinguish between types of databases

In the previous chapters, we have discussed principles of data collection, validity and measurements. In this chapter, we will focus on the principles of data management. Data management includes:

- Defining variables
- Creating database and data dictionary
- Entering data and rectifying errors
- Creating dataset for analysis, backing up and archiving dataset

17.1 ELEMENTS OF DATA MANAGEMENT

The key elements of data management are depicted in Figure 17.1.

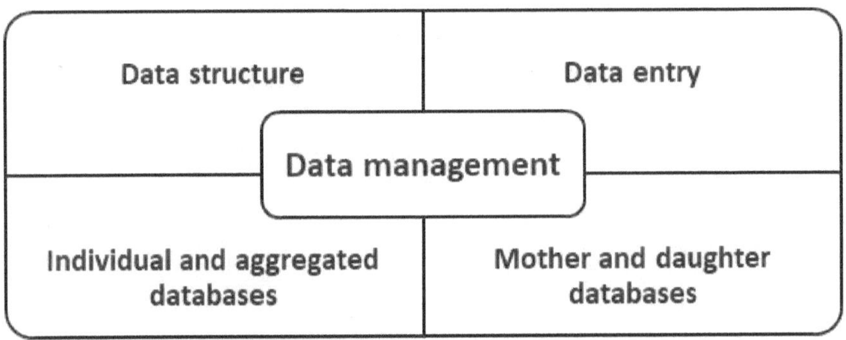

▲ **Figure 17.1:** Key elements of data management

17.1.1 Data Structure

Table 17.1 provides the structure of a database. A database is an organised collection of information generally stored and accessed electronically through a computer system. It usually contains several rows that represent records of individuals and columns that represent variables collected based on the study questions.

▼ **Table 17.1:** Structure of a database

	Identifier	Variable 1	Variable 2	Variable 3	Variable 4	Variable 5
Record 1						
Record 2						
Record 3						
Record 4						

Data Documentation

Data documentation is the mechanism of formulating a plan for data management. It includes information about the origin of the database in terms of its date of creation and modification, and a data structure containing the names, number of records, variables with coded values and storage-related information. It also includes information about the media in which data is stored, the mechanism of backing up the data and other relevant information.

Unique Identifier

The first important element of a database is the identifier. This identifier has to be unique for every participant. A computerised index system maintains it. The unique identifier has to be secured by a quality assurance procedure that guarantees that each data has internal validity. Unique identifiers are expressed as codes and can have several digits. A code comprises information about a particular participant. Each of the digits or set of digits in the code can refer to specific identification information about the participant.

Figure 17.2 shows the use of codes in a unique identifier. In the example, the first and second digits denote the village/area. The third and fourth digits represent the street name. The fifth digit indicates the house, apartment or residence door number. The last two digits denote the person's identification number. This seven-digit number would be unique for each participant.

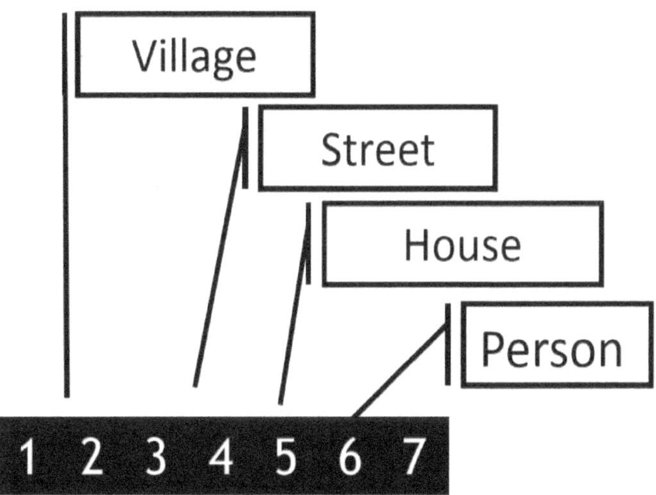

▲ **Figure 17.2:** Example of a code within a unique identifier

Structure of Variables in a Database

Right from the beginning of the study, researchers need to pay attention to different variables included in the study. They should specify whether the variable is an integer or a numeric; for integers, they should specify the number of digits. For numeric, they should mention the number of decimals accepted in the study. Additionally, they should note the length of the variable. It is advisable to use upper case (capital letters) for all the letters used in the variables to avoid errors while entering the data as both text and number. Finally, the researcher can also decide on a specific format for dates. The structure of the variables should include all these specifications.

Creating Variable Names

The first important point regarding data management is to have a clear idea about the data collection instrument while creating variable names. Each variable name should refer to an item mentioned in the questionnaire, and it has to be in an understandable format. For example, if the questionnaire item is about 'exercising': asking whether the individual exercises daily or not, the variable name could be 'EXERDAILY', which denotes what questionnaire item it refers to.

The second criterion is that the variable name should be kept short and without any space between the letters. Most software accept a maximum of ten characters only. Therefore, the variable names should be crisp and self-explanatory.

The third important aspect is that the variable names should be consistent. For example, let us consider different responses to a question on "how frequently somebody exercises". Exercising daily in the past can be denoted using the variable name, 'EXERPAST'. This is self-explanatory in its relationship to the particular questionnaire item. If the response is "currently exercising daily", then the variable could be 'EXERCURRDLY'; if the response is "occasionally exercised in the past", the variable name could be 'EXERPASTOCC'. In this manner, variable names should be framed such that, by looking at the variable name, the investigator can quickly identify the questionnaire item that it relates to.

Variable names can be given as a whole in situations where the responses are dichotomised. These are known as crude variables. For example, if a question relates to the number of times a participant exercises, the answer could be three times, four times, or five times a day. The researcher can divide the responses into two categories, namely 'exercised' and 'not exercised'. In this case, the researcher can assign 'EXERCISE' as a crude variable name. They can then change the variable name to EXERCISE_12, where the responses are dichotomised into 'exercised' (marked as 1) or 'not exercised' (marked as 2). However, the variable name should be consistent. The researcher must assign variable names for all responses. If a variable name is not assigned, the software will assign a variable name by itself, which can create confusion, including duplicates of similar items.

Design Data Entry-Friendly Data Collection Tool

Another critical factor to be kept in mind while creating data collection tools is to make them data entry-friendly. If the research goes on for long, another researcher may have to take over the data collection process. Hence, the data collection tool should be designed in an unambiguous manner. It should be divided into broad sections and then split into smaller sections. The researcher has to segregate the questionnaire responses into these sections when feeding them into a database at a later stage. For example, there could be a section called 'Identifier', which could be a unique ID, and another section called 'Demographics', which includes details about participants' age, gender, community and family-related information. The following section could be called 'Outcomes', and could collect information about the problem or disease in question. Information about other variables and potential confounders could be collected under a section titled, 'Exposures'.

Finally, the data collection tool should have an auto-coding option. If a researcher collects information on 'daily exercise' in the format of 'yes' or 'no', the responses should be entered in the database as 1 or 2. This is known as auto-coding. Therefore, data collection instruments should be designed in a way that allows effortless data entry.

Coding

Another important aspect of data entry is coding. It is always preferable to have numerical coding for quantitative studies. However, if textual information is collected in qualitative data, it should be coded differently. The researcher should also decide on the code to be used for missing values. It could be in the form of a dot (.) or 999 or 9,999 or 9,99,999 depending on the field chosen to enter. But one must be careful while coding for missing values. For example, one should not enter the missing value for age as 99.

For the 'Not applicable' response, you should use a specific code consistently throughout the instrument. If your data collectors are beginners who do not have much experience in handling databases, it is advisable not to create cumbersome regulations. This advice is applicable for senior researchers also. For example, for the question, "Do you walk every day?", 'walking' could be the variable coded as 1 (Yes) and 0 (No). For the question, "Do you cycle every day?", 'cycling' could be the variable coded as 1 (Yes) and 0 (No). However, if the next question is, "Do you do both walking and cycling?" and if the response to this question is Yes, the answer to this question should be coded as 1 (Yes) and 0 (No). The researcher should not confuse the response with '12'.

Another critical issue while using dichotomised variables is to code accurately. Code "1 for Yes" and "0 for No" or "1 for Yes" and "2 for No" or "1 for Present" and "2 for Absent" as a baseline for dichotomised variables. Different software can have different understanding of coding. Some may prefer "1 and 0" while others may use "1 and 2" during analysis. Hence, you need to be well aware about how your software works.

Constructing a Data Dictionary

Finally, a researcher needs to have a catalogue related to data entry. Before initiating data entry, researchers have to create a data dictionary or variable record that describes all variables related to the questionnaire items. The data dictionary should detail the values that will be assigned to the variables and the meaning of each value in a specific format (Table 17.2).

▼ **Table 17.2:** Structure of a data dictionary

Question	Variable name	Type	Format	Values	Logical checks
1	EXERDAILY	Integer	Yes No	=1 =2	Skip pattern
2	EXERTYPE	Integer	Walking Cycling	=1 =2	
ETC...					

Some software can generate data dictionary as a variable catalogue. However, researchers should develop their own data dictionary for the study, specifying the question item, variable name, type of a variable, data format and the collected data with logical checks, if required. Important details regarding study variables like operational definitions, coding, etc. should be given explicitly in the data dictionary. This will help subsequent researchers to work with the database without any confusion. It will also help the researcher keep a record of what has already been done and how it was done.

17.1.2 Data Entry

Before initiating data entry, researchers should double-check the numbers to be used in the data entry software to ensure internal validity. They have to mention the minimum and maximum values that can be entered in a particular field. For example, if the study is on children below five years of age, the age column should not accept any number above 5. This will help minimise errors during data entry.

The researcher should also specify skip patterns. Example: If one of the questions is "Do you exercise?" and the response of a participant is 'No', there should be an option to skip questions about the 'type of exercise', 'frequency of exercise', 'nature of exercise' and 'intensity of exercise', as they are not relevant based on the participant's response to the main question.

The researcher should also use automatic coding wisely. When a researcher is entering a code into a software, the code will automatically denote the corresponding response referred to in the data collection instrument. The researcher may need a certain amount of time to copy data from a preceding record. A code can do this automatically. For example, if laboratory results must be carried forward to another section, there may be a provision to reproduce the results automatically to the specified place in the database.

Further, calculations based on formulae can be done by the database itself. The researcher may only need to enter the values of the variables used in the calculations. For example, you may collect height and weight data. But you may not need to calculate the body mass index (BMI) in the data collection instrument. The database can do it—when the height and weight are entered, it can automatically calculate BMI if programmed accordingly.

Data Cleaning

The data entry process is an opportunity for data cleaning. While entering data into the database, it should be cleaned simultaneously. For example, researchers must provide clarifications or notes, if any, to the data entry person before data entry is commenced. The data entry person can also refer these notes to the investigator for additional inputs to clean up the data. Researchers can add automated data checks that will validate the data when it is being entered into the database. To prevent duplicate entries, it is advisable to mark each questionnaire after its data entry is completed.

17.1.3 Individual and Aggregated Databases

Databases can be individual or aggregated. The database that was described previously is individual or separate. Each 'record' in a row of a database is an observation. Aggregated databases are a compilation of several individual databases, where data will be entered as '*counts*' in each of the records. When only one count is entered, it is called a **normalised database.** A normalised database is one in which each row contains only one count for an individual record. For example, Table 17.3 below shows individual and aggregated databases. An individual database is shown on the left-hand side, wherein data about participants are entered according to their place of residence, age, sex and onset of disease. Each of the rows is an 'individual'. Using such individual databases, we can create an aggregated database. As shown on the right of Table 17.3, a researcher can retrieve the number of participants affected by the disease, sorted according to place of residence.

▼ **Table 17.3:** Individual and aggregated database showing participants' demographic details

Individual data

ID	Place	Age	Sex	Onset
1	A	3	1	1 Jan 06
2	B	1	2	1 Jan 06
3	C	35	2	3 Jan 06
4	D	67	1	4 Jan 06
5	A	2	1	2 Jan 06
6	B	2	1	4 Jan 06
7	C	2	1	5 Jan 06

Aggregated data of people with disease

ID	Place	Count
1	A	5
2	B	3
3	C	37
4	D	67

Note: A, B, C and D are the codes used for denoting place of residence.

17.1.4 Mother and Daughter Databases

There are two other variants of databases called mother and daughter databases. Data may be collected at various levels like district, village, household or individual classes in a study. Information can also be collected personally about several episodes of illness. Therefore, a researcher may gather different levels of information during data collection. But it is not necessary to repeat the same details in every section of the record. For example, if a researcher collects information about village and household levels, it is not necessary to repeat village details while entering the household details. The researcher can keep the two databases separate at their levels and link them as required, at the time of data analysis. For example, Table 17.4 shows individual and household level data. The household level data has information about the house identification number (ID) (as 1, 2, 3, 4, 5 etc.), location (as A, B, C, D, E and F), community code and status of household income (coded as 1, 2, etc.). In the individual level dataset, we have house ID (corresponding to the ID used in the household database), personal identification number (ID), status of disease (coded) and status of exposure (coded).

All the coding used in all the databases should be described clearly in the data collection instrument. We can see here that the house ID is repeated in both databases. The person ID is the identity of individuals in the included households. The two databases were created separately. Each database has its own unique identifier, and multiple databases can be linked using a standard index identifier. Here, the two databases can be linked using the common variable, household ID, with the help of any statistical software.

▼ **Table 17.4:** Two databases showing household level and individual level database

Household level data

House ID	Location	Community	Household income
1	A	3	1
2	B	1	2
3	C	35	2
4	D	67	1
5	E	2	1
6	F	2	1

Individual level data

House ID	Person ID	Diseased	Exposed
1	101	1	1
1	102	2	1
2	201	2	2
2	202	1	2

In data management, you need to code databases numerically, enter data by following quality assurance procedures, store information and relate or merge files.

References and Further Reading

1. Den AG, Arner TG, Sunki GG, Friedman R, Latinga M, Sangam S et al. Epi Info™, a database and statistics program for public health professionals. Atlanta, GA, USA: CDC; 2011.
2. Link to Epi Info software https://www.cdc.gov/epiinfo/support/downloads.html.
3. Krishnankutty B, Bellary S, Kumar NB, Moodahadu LS. Data management in clinical research: an overview. *Indian J Pharmacol.* 2012; 44 (2):168-72.
4. Surkis A, Read K. Research data management. *J Med LibrAssoc.*2015;103(3):154-6.

CHAPTER 18

OVERVIEW OF DATA ANALYSIS

P. Manickam

Learning Objectives

At the end of this chapter, readers will be able to:

1. Describe the sequence of data analysis strategy
2. Relate plan of analysis to the nature of research question
3. Outline the steps for initial and advanced stages of analysis

The essence of research is to link an exposure to an outcome. Therefore, we analyse data to measure the impact of a clinical or public health programme, address the chance of error, bias, and other potential confounding factors, and ultimately assess the causality of exposure and outcome.

18.1 SEQUENCE OF DATA ANALYSIS STRATEGY

There is a specific sequence for performing data analysis. The strategy of data analysis can be divided into seven steps:

1. Identify the study type
2. Identify the main variables
3. Familiarise yourself with the data
4. Characterise the study population
5. Examine the association between exposure and outcome
6. Create additional two-way tables
7. Conduct advanced analysis

18.1.1 Identify Study Type

Identifying the study type is the first and foremost step that researchers should do before starting data analysis. Researchers must decide whether they are dealing with a descriptive or an analytical study design. In case of a descriptive study, they need to estimate the frequency of the disease and calculate appropriate indicators, such as incidence or prevalence. In case of an analytical study, they must test the hypotheses using appropriate statistical tests.

The plan for analysing research data primarily depends on the study objectives and study design. Therefore, the research question must be stated clearly, mentioning whether the study is only a descriptive study that is conducted in a group for estimating a quantity, or if it is an analytical study that involves the comparison of two groups or intervention for testing a hypothesis. Depending on the study design, researchers can select the data analysis plan. In the case of a descriptive study, wherein the researchers are describing only a group of people, they should specify whether the outcome of interest is acute or chronic.

Depending on the outcome of interest, appropriate measures of disease frequency should be applied. For descriptive studies: Incidence is reported for acute diseases and prevalence is measured for chronic diseases. For analytical studies: If the study outcome is acute and the outcome of interest is frequently occurring, as in diarrhoea or acute respiratory tract infections, a cohort study would be an ideal design to use. In this case, relative risk or risk ratio (RR) is an appropriate measure of association. If the occurrence of the disease is rare, a case-control study would be ideal. In such a case, odds ratio (OR) should be used as the measure of association.

However, if the disease outcome is chronic (for example, non-communicable diseases like carcinoma or diabetes), a prevalent case-control study will be a suitable study design. In this case, the prevalence odds ratio (POR) will be an appropriate measure of association. In an analytical cross-sectional study designed to analyse chronic and frequently-occurring diseases (like hypertension and road traffic accident), prevalence ratio is the preferred measure of association. Thus, the data analysis plan depends on the research question and the study design.

18.1.2 Identify Main Variables

The second step of data analysis is identifying the main study variables. The study should explicitly identify the exposure(s), outcome variable(s) and potential covariates in the study protocol. Furthermore, variables for additional analysis (such as subgroup analysis) should be described clearly in the protocol.

18.1.3 Familiarise Yourself With the Data

The third step of data analysis is familiarising oneself with the data. First, the frequency distribution of the variables and the findings should be closely examined by looking at the distribution of the variables. Then, some descriptive analysis has to be done for the study population. This will give the researcher a good overview of the data. Second, the number of observations across the variables **need to be reviewed** to identify any duplicates or missing values. Then, the observations and entries should be cross-checked for acceptable and logical values, against the values mentioned in the data dictionary. The consistency in the pattern of the data should also be checked simultaneously. Familiarising oneself with the data is crucial, and so researchers should spend sufficient time in this step.

18.1.4 Characterise the Study Population

The fourth step of data analysis is to characterise the study population in terms of socio-demographic and economic variables, such as age, gender, education, occupation and income groups. However, if the study involves control groups, the distribution of the study population across the variables should be observed to determine the comparability among the groups. Additionally, the frequency of occurrence of clinical features of the disease in the people should be observed closely. This will give the researcher an idea about the occurrence and pattern of the disease in the population.

18.1.5 Examine the Association Between Exposure and Outcome

The fifth step of data analysis is to examine the association between outcome and exposure. This is the most exciting phase of data analysis and is based on *a priori* (before the analysis) hypotheses. In this step, researchers compare the frequency of exposure in two or more groups using appropriate measures of association, based on prior knowledge about the variables. Each study design has its own measurement of association for a specific type of exposure and outcome. For example, in a case-control study, the strength of association between exposure and outcome is expressed as the odds ratio (OR). In a cohort study, the measure of association is risk ratio (RR).

Additionally, to compensate for potential confounding factors, researchers perform appropriate analyses at various stages of the study. For example, in the design stage of an epidemiological study, researchers may apply matching or restriction of variables depending on the study design. Whereas, in the analysis stage of a study, researchers can apply appropriate stratified analysis, regression or multivariate analysis to compensate for potential confounding factors.

18.1.6 Create Additional Two-Way Tables

The sixth step of data analysis is to create a two-way table for analysing new variables that may be detected in the findings of the study. Researchers can do this by stating the newly created variables, mentioning how they were created and explaining how they should be analysed.

18.1.7 Conduct Advanced Analysis

The seventh and final step of data analysis is to conduct some advanced analysis based on the requirement of your research objective. This could be a dose-response effect analysis, stratification analysis or multivariate modelling analysis.

18.2 SOME PRACTICAL TIPS FOR DATA ANALYSIS

There are some valuable tips that every researcher should keep in mind while performing data analysis. These are grouped below according to the steps of data analysis.

18.2.1 Prior Plan for Data Analysis

The plan for data analysis should be prepared in advance. Researchers should create dummy tables for analysis even before starting the analysis. They should review the study objective, study design (such as cross-sectional, case-control or cohort etc.), measures of disease frequency (incidence or prevalence) and the proposed measures of association (odds ratio, risk/rate ratio or prevalence ratio) to prepare the dummy tables. Then, they should prepare a list of dummy tables required to meet the study objectives. They should be cautious to avoid duplication of data and should be clear about the variables to be used in the data analysis. They can also use checklists from standard guidelines (for example, those available at https://www.equator-network.org/) to prepare the data analysis plan.

18.2.2 Initial Stages of Data Analysis

During the initial stages of data analysis, researchers must look at the exposure and outcome variables and recode the variables if required. They should also create new variables from the existing ones or categorise the current variables based on the need (vide infra), if required.

Qualitative variables should be dichotomised, i.e., categorised as 'Yes' and 'No'. For example, suppose the objective of a research study is, "to measure the effect of brisk walking on fasting blood sugar levels in diabetics". Here, the outcome is reduced blood sugar levels: yes (1) and no (0).

Continuous variables can be recoded into groups. For example, age can be categorised as 25–34 years, 35–44 years, 45–54 years, 55–64 years and so on. Similarly, income can be categorised into quartiles or socioeconomic scales. For example, the modified Kuppuswamy scale classifies socioeconomic status into five categories—upper, upper-middle, lower-middle, upper-lower and lower. Here is another example: 'exercise' can be classified as mild, moderate, heavy or no exercise. The researcher can create groups in the recording stage and, during the descriptive phase, calculate the outcome frequency for each of these groups. This is a sequential process that researchers should follow without skipping.

18.2.3 Analytical Stage of Data Analysis

Data analysis can be done in three different ways. One way is a univariate analysis, wherein the outcome frequency is described using one variable only. For example, in the univariate analysis for the study mentioned above "to measure the effect of brisk walking on fasting blood sugar levels in diabetics", the frequency of the outcome of interest, "reduction of blood sugar level", can be expressed by age, gender, income and other variables.

The second way of performing data analysis is to conduct a stratified or dose-response analysis, through which the researcher can examine the outcome as per categories of a particular variable. For example, the researcher may wish to analyse the exposure, 'exercise', and its relationship with the outcome, 'reduction in blood sugar level' among participants, stratified according to age, gender and income. The third way of performing data analysis is using a logistic regression model. In the above example, this model can be used to determine whether exercise can reduce fasting blood sugar levels in people with diabetes.

18.2.4 Avoid Post-Hoc Analysis

Any analysis that was not included in the initial plan and is only driven by the collected data is called post-hoc analysis. Researchers should avoid doing any such post-hoc analysis of the data collected.

18.3 SOFTWARE FOR DATA MANAGEMENT AND ANALYSIS

For your research, it is preferable to use software that will provide data management and data analysis capabilities. For example, EpiInfo can create a data collection instrument, enter data, analyse data and map the information. It can also perform statistical analysis.

Data analysis should be planned during the initial phase of protocol preparation and must be explained in detail in the protocol to avoid any post-hoc analysis. Moreover, study analysis should be carried out stage by stage, as mentioned in this chapter.

References and Further Reading

1. ICMR School of Public Health. Sequence of data analysis strategy. ICMR-National Institute of Epidemiology, Chennai, India. (Appendix I)
2. ICMR School of Public Health. Dummy table shells for reports. ICMR-National Institute of Epidemiology, Chennai, India. (Appendix II)
3. Chapter 4 – Basic biostatistics: concepts and tools. In: Bonita R, Beaglehole R, Kjellstrom T. Basic epidemiology. 2nd ed. Geneva: World Health Organization; 2006: p. 63-82.

SECTION V

CONDUCTING A RESEARCH STUDY

ETHICAL FRAMEWORK FOR HEALTH RESEARCH

Sanjay Mehendale

Learning Objectives

At the end of this chapter, readers will be able to:

1. Identify the range of ethical issues that need to be addressed in health research
2. Describe the fundamental ethical principles involving human participants
3. List the key national and international guidelines and regulations that guide the development and review of research studies
4. Recognise the process and issues related to the conduct of health research and practice of medicine

Researchers must have a thorough knowledge about ethical issues to ensure the safety and welfare of the research participants. This chapter will give an overview about some of the important ethical issues that need to be considered in health and biomedical research.

19.1 ETHICAL FOUNDATION FOR RESEARCH

Remember that ethical foundation is considered implicit for conducting any research. It is applicable not only to health research but extends to research in general. Any research involving human participants should follow international standards of ethics. The Indian Council of Medical Research (ICMR), which is the apex body in India for the formulation, coordination and promotion of biomedical research, and one of the oldest medical research bodies in the world, has developed the Indian National Standards for ethics, that are on par with international guidelines. These guidelines are quintessential for conducting research.

There is a misconception among researchers that ethics review is required only in cases where significant risk is involved, such as while using invasive procedures. However, this is incorrect. As researchers, we need to remember that even when data is readily available and there is no risk to human participants, ethics review is required. Ethics review is also mandatory in situations when there is minimal risk such as, when participants are interviewed using a standard questionnaire and no samples or specimens are collected.

19.2 EVOLUTION OF GUIDELINES FOR PRACTICE OF ETHICS IN BIOMEDICAL RESEARCH

From the beginning of the 20th century, many international guidelines have been developed for improving ethical practices in biomedical research. During World War II, several unethical experiments were conducted on the captives. Numerous atrocities were committed upon human participants by using them for research in an unfair manner. At the end of the war, these inhumanities paved way for discussions on ethical conduct of research.

One such effort in this direction that began very early was the development of the **Nuremberg Code in 1947**. This code initiated discussions on the rationale and justification for conducting research on humans. It raised the question of "whether a particular research is necessary based on its importance". It advocates for the execution of a risk-benefit analysis that weighs the advantage that a participant might gain against the harm or detriment they might suffer if they participated in the study. It also provides guidelines for competence of investigators and importance of voluntary consent in research.

Thereafter, for the first time, many countries came together and signed a landmark document called **Helsinki Declaration** in 1964. This declaration has been revised several times since then and the latest revision was published in 2013. The Helsinki Declaration provides guidelines about individuals' right to make informed decisions, duties of investigators, patients' rights, research participants' welfare and protection of the interests of groups that are considered as vulnerable.

During 1978–79, the **Belmont report** was published in the United States of America, describing the basic ethical principles of autonomy, justice and beneficence. It also reemphasised the importance of informed consent in research. In addition, for the first time, the importance of a review by an ethics committee called Institutional Review Board was emphasised in the West.

In 1992–93, the Council of International Organization on Medical Sciences and the World Health Organization developed a document called

CIOMS guidelines, which was later revised in 2002. This document provides guidelines for reporting adverse drug reactions and threat to the safety of research participants. This is particularly relevant in clinical research and clinical trials, where new drugs and vaccines are tested on human participants. The CIOMS guidelines also explain about 'benefit and risk balance' and 'need and principles of pharmacovigilance'. The CIOMS guidelines is the first document that stressed that the responsibility of investigators goes beyond phase 1, 2 and 3 studies, to a continued surveillance of the population to learn about the long-term safety of their interventions.

In 1996, the **International Council on Harmonization**, or **ICH**, as it is popularly called, developed basic guidelines for good clinical practice. Subsequently, drawing basic rules from this document, the good clinical laboratory practice document and good clinical epidemiological practice document were developed. These documents have found applications in different spheres of health-related research.

19.3 ICMR—ETHICAL GUIDELINES FOR RESEARCH ON HUMAN PARTICIPANTS

India is not far behind in developing its own ethics guidelines. In 2000, ICMR introduced ethical guidelines for research on human participants. This was a major consensus document that was subsequently revised in 2006 and 2017. This document is available on the ICMR website. It provides ethical guidance for carrying out bio-medical or health research involving human beings, for all institutions across the country. It provides the guidelines that researchers have to follow to protect the safety and well-being of all individuals involved in their research.

In addition, there are several other national guidelines such as the document on **Genome policy and Genetic Research (2000)**, **Amendment of Drugs and Cosmetic Act (2002)**, guidelines for **Assisted Reproductive Technology (2005)**, and **Stem Cell Research and Bio-Banking (2006)**. Researchers working in these areas must be aware of these guidelines and adhere to them while conducting their respective research.

19.4 ETHICAL PRINCIPLES

There are four basic ethical principles that every researcher should strictly adhere to while conducting research: respect for autonomy, justice, beneficence and non-maleficence.

19.4.1 Autonomy

Autonomy is a Latin word for 'self-rule'. Researchers should respect individuals for who they are. They have an obligation to respect the decisions made by people concerning their own lives, which implies respecting their human dignity. They must not interfere with the decisions of competent adults such as what people feel like doing or people's thought processes. However, they must actively empower people who are not adequately aware or knowledgeable about a particular research. Autonomy means that people should be clearly informed that they have a right to decide whether to participate in a research or not.

19.4.2 Justice

Justice emphasises that researchers have an obligation to provide the population with whatever they deserve. They have an obligation to treat all people equally, fairly and impartially. The benefit of research should be extended to everybody except, in certain situations say, when pregnant women cannot participate in a certain research. Unless contraindicated, all groups should be given equal opportunity to participate in research. However, the researcher should never impose the research on participants in an unfair manner.

The next two principles go hand-in-hand.

19.4.3 Beneficence

Beneficence means that researchers must be fair and correct in all their actions. They must take positive steps to prevent harm. Sometimes, in the endeavour to pursue beneficence, researchers may place themselves in direct conflict with respecting the autonomy of people. This has to be avoided.

19.4.4 Non-Maleficence

Non-maleficence complements the principle of beneficence. "Do No Harm" is the principle behind non-maleficence. For example, when testing a new drug trial, there is always a chance of adverse effects. As researchers, whenever harm cannot be completely avoided, one needs to take appropriate measures to minimise harm. Besides, it is also wrong to waste resources that could be used for good.

19.5 INFORMED CONSENT

One of the ways of ensuring that ethical principles are adhered to is through a process called "Informed Consent". This is performed as a process since it is neither a one-time event nor a rule that can be satisfied with a tick mark. It is a systematic method in which the proposed research is explained to the potential participants in an orderly, step-by-step manner and the potential participants are empowered to take an informed decision to participate in the research study.

Informed consent includes the following rules. Participants must understand about the study procedures, the risks and benefits of their participation. They should know that they have the liberty to ask questions, raise concerns and have them appropriately answered by the researchers. Finally, the participants should take a learned and informed decision to either participate or not participate in the study.

It can take several sessions to complete this process. The participant may understand the whole process in one single sitting or may require multiple sittings and multiple sessions. Researchers have to persevere and take the potential participants through the process meticulously. In studies involving tribal populations or institutional setups, it is important to obtain a group consent or consent from the concerned authorities. However, one should remember that although group consent is desirable, it cannot replace individual consent.

19.6 INFORMED CONSENT DOCUMENT

Informed consent is an appeal or invitation to participate in a research, written in simple, easy to understand, local language. The Informed Consent document should have a header with the name of the project and the agency that is conducting the research.

The main body of the document should contain the following details. It should contain the **research description** in brief. It should explain the **potential risks** and **benefits**. It has to explain whether the research will benefit the participating individual or the community as a whole. The **alternatives to not participating** in the research must also be explained. For example, participants must be explained that they will continue to get the services that they would otherwise get, even if they decide not to participate in the study. When sensitive information is collected, participants may be worried about the safety of such information. Therefore, researchers have to commit and give an **assurance of confidentiality**, guaranteeing that the participants' records will be kept confidential. If a participant is harmed in any way due to their participation in the research, they have to be appropriately **compensated**. A clause to this respect should be included in the informed consent document.

Researchers should also provide the contact information of the person(s) whom the research participants can contact to obtain any additional information or clarify any concerns that they may have about the study. In addition, one important clause that is added is about **voluntary participation**. The informed consent document must specify that every person has a right to decide whether to participate or not participate in the research. This is especially important in case of a long-term follow-up study. The document should explain that, if a person decides to **drop out of the study** at any point of time, it is perfectly within the rights of the individual to do so. At the end of the informed consent document, the signature of the participant and if the participant is an illiterate, then the signature of a witness who is not a part of the study team has to be obtained.

19.7 STAKEHOLDERS IN THE INFORMED CONSENT PROCESS

In research, informed consent is an inevitable procedure. There are several stakeholders involved in the informed consent process, like researchers, institutions, participants, sponsors, monitors and regulators.

Researchers and research institutions are obliged to provide in-depth information about the research to the participants. The participants should be given a chance to discuss their issues and concerns, and be provided with adequate explanation. Researchers should also ensure that the participants have adequately understood the information about the research and ensure that they take a voluntary decision to participate. There should be no coercion or coaxing on the part of the researchers.

Study participants have to fully understand the information provided to them about the research study. They should not sign the informed consent form without understanding the purpose, procedure and other clauses in the study. They have to be aware of their rights and understand the provisions written in the informed consent document. They should sign the consent form independently and without any coercion or force.

The sponsors, monitors and regulators have the authority to assess the fairness of the consenting process at various levels. The institutional ethics committee will begin this assessment prior to the approval of the research study and continue monitoring the entire procedure. They also have the authority to verify the consent documentation of the research participants. Thence, each and every stakeholder involved in the research has a unique and combined responsibility to ensure that the informed consent is appropriately obtained.

19.8 ISSUES RELATED TO INFORMED CONSENT

There are some questions that are commonly raised while administering the informed consent form. These are answered in detail below.

"Whom does the informed consent benefit?"

It benefits both the participants as well as the researcher. From the participants' point of view, it provides them with the required information to aid in independent decision making. From the investigator's perspective, it is a valid documentation that proves that the informed consent process has been completed in the most appropriate manner.

"Are the research procedure and other aspects of research adequately explained in the informed consent form?"

To ensure a better understanding, consent forms are written in the local language, with simple and clear information. To test the accuracy of the translation, the consent form is first translated into the local language, then back-translated into English and then certified and order-checked with the original English consent form. This is called linguistic validation. Besides this, investigators also conduct a 'test of understanding', which is a good practice. The 'test of understanding' is a small objective-type test that is given to the research participants after they sign the informed consent form, to quickly assess whether their understanding of the form is adequate.

"Who can be a witness to the consent procedure?"

A witness is required when participants are illiterate and so cannot sign the informed consent form. In such instances, there needs to be an impartial witness, who is a literate but not a part of the research team. This witness should sign the form on behalf of the participant.

"Can there be different types of informed consent?"

There has been a lot of discussion about whether oral consent is valid or not. Oral consent is valid only in case of exceptional circumstances and should be approved by the ethics committee as per the National Ethical Guidelines for Biomedical and Health Research involving Human Participants (2017). Typically, participants have to sign two copies of the informed consent form, out of which one will be returned back to them. They can retain this copy with themselves for record since it would contain answers to questions that might arise in their mind any time later, during the research. There has been some hue and cry about the need for audio and visual consent. The regulatory authorities in India have now made it mandatory to record the consent procedures for studies involving Investigational New Drugs (IND) in India. This is an important regulation that researchers must bear in mind while conducting research.

19.9 IMPORTANCE OF SCIENTIFIC REVIEW

Scientific and regulatory reviews need to be conducted prior to ethics review and before implementing a study. Scientific review looks at the novelty, rationality and relevance of the study. It validates the justification for conducting the study in the context of national priorities, the scientific merits of the research project and its feasibility such as review of toxicological studies, laboratory and animal data, technology transfer and capacity building at sites. It also examines the soundness of the study design extensively. It verifies whether appropriate study procedures have been taken into consideration, the inclusion and exclusion criteria, whether the sample size has been calculated appropriately, the randomisation and blinding procedures if any, how the end-points or outcomes will be assessed, the follow-up schedule, the pharmacy plan, and the investigator responsibilities to the participants beyond the study. A thorough scientific review is important since well-planned research studies are more likely to correctly address human participants' ethical issues.

19.10 OBJECTIVES OF REGULATORY REVIEW

Regulatory reviews evaluate **pre-clinical trial data**, which is data about the clinical trials related to the study topic, that were previously conducted. This is particularly important in case of new drugs and new vaccines. Regulatory reviews also perform the **in-country regulatory assessments** that are specially applicable for **drugs, vaccines and product imports**. This is important in the case of trials that use products that were developed outside the country. These assessments ensure that the national requirements for special scenarios, such as the use of genetically engineered products, stem cell research, research on reproductive technologies, organ transplantation, etc. are properly met.

Sample shipment and transfers as well as transfer of raw data are monitored very seriously by the Government of India. There are also issues of intellectual property rights in this field. So, researchers are expected to know these issues and regulations fairly well in this regard. Adherence to restrictions regarding the exchange of scientists and visitors is also verified in this review. Budget, foreign funding in particular, is a domain that comes under regulatory review. Researchers conducting studies in the country border or high-security areas have to be aware of the regulatory requirements in such situations. Similar to a scientific review, a carefully performed regulatory review also helps in answering some ethical concerns.

19.11 ETHICAL ISSUES

The following are the ethical issues that need to be addressed while conducting a health research. It is necessary to assess the competence of the researchers and the research team in conducting the research. Provisions for the protection of human rights and ethical issues, especially for vulnerable populations, women and children in particular, have to be addressed. Measures taken by the researcher to protect the confidentiality of the individual participants and avoid discrimination must be stated. Appropriateness and completeness of the informed consent form and study-specific educational material has to be evaluated. Mechanisms for reporting and managing adverse events and serious adverse events should be in place. This is particularly important in case of drug trials.

Care and support mechanism for participants, including the standard of care provided, long-term care and post-trial access to care and products, if any, should be specified. This section should also mention whether medical support would be extended to the participants after the trial, whether post-trial benefits would be given to the community after the trial and whether it would prove to be useful. These aspects should also be looked at from an ethics perspective. Reimbursements and compensation are also important considerations that need to be verified while conducting ethics review. The researcher has to ensure that the participants are reimbursed for the time lost and expenses incurred for traveling to the clinical research site. While compensation is usually given in case of unforeseen injury that arises due to the research, incentives may be given to encourage participation in the research. However, the reimbursements, compensation and incentives should not be so much, as to force people to participate in the research trial. This aspect has to be reviewed by the ethics committee. The regulatory authorities should continue to review the progress of the study until its completion.

19.12 RESPONSIBILITY OF INSTITUTIONAL ETHICS COMMITTEES OR INSTITUTIONAL REVIEW BOARD

The committee that looks at a proposed research from an ethics standpoint is called the Institutional Ethics Committee or Institutional Review Board. These committees keenly scrutinise the proposed study's real or potential, and individual or community benefit, whether there is adequate protection of the rights of research participants, whether the potential benefits of the study outweigh the risks associated with research participation, whether the participants and communities will have access to study findings and benefits of research, and the mechanisms for providing safety, care and support to research participants during and after the study.

19.13 ETHICS INFLUENCING HEALTH RESEARCH AND PRACTICE OF MEDICINE

In recent times, there are growing expectations about accountability from researchers. Researchers are now being questioned about their responsibility and that of the government in conducting research in a fair manner. Advocacy movements have increased public awareness about medical research. All this will eventually help in improving the quality of research and influencing the practice of medicine in due course of time.

In today's world, there is a collective demand for health benefits. People are demanding 'universal right to healthcare', which emanates from the principle of 'health for all'. This leads to the demand that more research have to be undertaken to make more benefits available to the common man.

Although researchers have the responsibility to follow ethics, research participants too have to fulfil certain expectations. The onus is also on self-responsibility, rather than blaming researchers for mishaps. Participants have to adapt the recommended lifestyle and follow appropriately whatever is expected of them, as explained in the informed consent form.

In recent times, following ethics in the practice of public health and health research is being increasingly addressed. We know that there are challenges as well, with ever-increasing public expectations and demands. Therefore, the search for solutions should be an ongoing process. To achieve this, various stakeholders such as the public health system, policymakers, researchers and program managers should show enough sensitivity and realise that there is scope for further improvement.

References and Further Reading

1. Indian Council of Medical Research. National ethical guidelines for biomedical and health research involving human participants. New Delhi: ICMR; 2017. https://ethics.ncdirindia.org//asset/pdf/Handbook_on_ICMR_Ethical_Guidelines.pdf
2. Council for International Organizations of Medical Sciences (CIOMS). International Ethical Guidelines for Biomedical Research Involving Human Participants Geneva: WHO, CIOMS; 2016. https://cioms.ch/wp-content/uploads/2017/01/WEB-CIOMS-EthicalGuidelines.pdf

CONDUCTING CLINICAL TRIALS

Sanjay Mehendale

Learning Objectives

At the end of this chapter, readers will be able to:

1. Recognise the importance of various reviews prior to the implementation of clinical trials
2. Identify critical issues in trial implementation

20.1 SCENARIO OF CLINICAL TRIALS IN INDIA

Clinical trials in India have gone through a lot of changes over the last 25 to 30 years. Although research institutes and the pharmaceutical industry have been performing clinical trials since the late 20th century, they were limited in nature. Since the first decade of the 21st century, the number of clinical trials being conducted in India began increasing. However, in the present decade, it is facing some challenges due to the regulatory reforms that were introduced in 2012–13.

International investigators and sponsors who wish to conduct high-quality clinical trials perceive that there are certain challenges in conducting clinical trials in India. They feel that ethical and regulatory **approvals are often delayed in India**. They also have concerns about the **quality of ethical review** since only in the recent times, systematic effort is being taken to improve the performance of various ethics committees, particularly in research organisations. The **shipment of samples (both import and export)** and **the transfer of data** are other concerns of international investigators as the Government of India has specific restrictions and regulations regarding the transfer of data and samples. They also perceive a deficiency **in trained investigators and centres** for conducting quality research.

The clause related to compensation for trial participants and recording of consent is a new regulatory reform that was recently introduced. The office of the Drug Controller General of India has given specific recommendations for calculating the compensation and the period until which these laws are applicable. This issue has been pressurising the researchers conducting clinical trials. However, there is still a lack of clear understanding of this particular topic among researchers.

Audio-visual recording of the informed consent process will help ensure accountability and transparency throughout the entire research process. If researchers protect the confidentiality of the trial participants adequately, audio-visual recording is the best possible proof of the efficacy of the consent procedure. Audio-visual recording is currently a requirement for IND trials (Investigational New Drug trials), which are also perceived as a challenge to be conducted in India by the international community.

20.2 SCIENTIFIC, ETHICAL AND REGULATORY REVIEWS

For all clinical trials, it is mandatory to get scientific, ethical and regulatory approvals. A scientific review looks at whether the research question is sound and whether every step of the study is described in detail. The Institutional Scientific Advisory Committee decides whether the proposed study design is appropriate and accurate. Once the scientific committee approves the study, the proposal must be submitted for **ethics review**. The Institutional Ethics Committee conducts the ethics review. At the national level, the ethics review is conducted by the National Ethics Committee. The ethics committee checks whether the safety and welfare of the research participants are adequately protected in the study. This is a critical aspect of clinical trials since there is an added necessity to abide by the ethical principle 'to not harm' research participants when they participate in the study.

Regulatory review is another mandate for conducting a clinical trial, which examines whether the research methods are appropriate. For interventional trials on new drugs, the Drug Controller General of India and currently the Standards Control Organisation are the regulatory bodies. If a project is receiving international funding, then the Health Ministry Screening Committee reviews the regulations around it. If the research study involves genetically modified or engineered products, the Genetic Engineering Approval Committee has to approve the study. It is the responsibility of the sponsors and investigators/researchers to find out about the regulatory approvals required for clinical trials in a particular context. All the mentioned approvals must be obtained before initiating the study. The approvals must be kept safe and ready for review by external monitors or other authorised agencies.

20.3 ADDRESSING ETHICAL ISSUES IN CLINICAL TRIALS

In a clinical trial, the researcher manipulates the environment. Hence, there is potential for several ethical issues to arise during the study, which need to be addressed. The following are some of the problems that might arise and strategies for addressing them. There should be a mechanism in place for conducting independent ethical review. Researchers should seek for necessary approvals from the ethics committee and in-country regulatory authorities as per the norm applicable in the country of study. After initial approval by the ethics committee, there should be mechanisms in place to ensure the protection of human participants throughout the trial. Adequate community engagement and support should be obtained. This is because, there have been instances when researchers were unaware of the interventions that were culturally unacceptable, leading to backlashes from the community. Hence, it is always necessary to obtain the support of stakeholders from the community, private practitioners, programme managers, politicians, local leaders and caretakers of the study participants.

It is mandatory to get informed consent from every participant before commencing a trial. Even after the trial is completed, the responsibility of the researchers does not end. While planning the research protocol, they should set up a mechanism for providing follow-up care and post-trial support to the participants.

The use of placebos in trials has raised some concerns in the past. However, using placebos is justified in the case of interventional vaccine or drug trials wherein the absence of a comparable vaccine or drug is accepted as the standard of care for a particular disease. Another important ethical issue is ensuring **the confidentiality of the study participants**. The study participants may not be comfortable disclosing their participation in the research even to their kith and kin. Therefore, the investigators or researchers must protect the participants' interests and ensure that the information collected is kept confidential.

20.4 CRITICAL ISSUES IN TRIAL IMPLEMENTATION

One of the crucial considerations in clinical trial implementation is the **Informed Consent procedure.** The word 'procedure' has been deliberately used here. The term 'Informed' implies that the researchers should explain the study procedure to the participants in detail. They should also ensure that any questions or concerns raised by the participants are adequately addressed. The participants may or may not understand the information provided to them in a single sitting and may require multiple sittings. This must be entertained and accommodated by the researcher. Once the participant understands the provided information, they should sign the consent form in the presence of an impartial witness who is not a member of the research team. A duplicate copy of the signed form containing the study information should be given to the participants to enable them to clarify any doubts that arise later. The investigators should retain another copy with themselves for safe documentation.

The process of clinical trial participation happens in two steps: screening and enrolment. During screening, **as per the protocol**, individuals interested in participating in the trial must undergo an assessment, which involves an interview followed by a medical examination and a sample collection specific to the study. The researchers should ensure that the participants fit into the eligibility criteria by strictly adhering to the inclusion and exclusion criteria mentioned in the protocol.

Researchers should follow **acceptable clinical and laboratory practices** throughout the trial. Study procedures, including the enrolment of study participants, collection of samples and frequency of visits should be strictly followed as described in the protocol. Quality control mechanisms should be in place and investigators and sponsors should ensure proper quality assurance. Researchers should also devise means for ensuring participant **adherence to intervention and follow-up**. In drug trials, they have to ensure that the patient takes the drug regularly.

Similarly, in follow-up studies, researchers have to ensure that the participant appears for follow-up at the defined time intervals. For example, a researcher wants to conduct a vaccine trial for preventing malaria by examining the immunogenicity potential of a particular vaccine for two years from the date of administration. If there is more than one dose to the vaccine, the researcher should ensure that the enrolled participants receive all the doses at pre-defined intervals. Then, the researcher should periodically monitor the serum antibody levels in the participants, say once every three months, for two years after administering the vaccine. The researcher must ensure that measures are in place to conduct follow-up every three months and collect blood samples from the participants. If patients miss some of these visits, the researcher will likely miss important information about them, such as the presence and levels of antibodies in their bodies at various time periods.

Multicentric trials are conducted in multiple sites within and across countries. In such cases, the researchers may find it difficult to gather the required number of participants for the study in certain areas. This can seriously compromise the quality of the research due to variations in following procedures among various centres. Hence, standardisation of the study protocols, training the research team before implementing the study and periodic retraining of the research team are essential.

One of the important prerequisites for conducting clinical trials is the presence of an **independent monitoring mechanism**. The sponsor for the study should employ an agency for monitoring the study independently with an objective, unbiased outlook. This agency should monitor the clinical practices followed, dispensing of study products, record maintenance, informed consent procedure, etc.

Since the safety of the participants is of paramount importance, **safety assessments** are built into all clinical trials. There should be well-defined reporting mechanisms for managing adverse and severely adverse events that may occur among the clinical trial participants. These events should be reported in a timely manner to the regulatory authorities, sponsors and ethics committees. Adverse events may be clinical issues, odd laboratory values or even social or familial problems that participants face while participating in the clinical trial. All information regarding such adverse events should be properly recorded and documented.

The next crucial consideration in a clinical trial is the **reimbursements** to be given to the trial participants to compensate for the time spent by them for the study, their loss of daily wages, travel costs to reach the study site and food expenses incurred. Reimbursements are provided mainly in the case of trials that require the study participants' long-term cooperation. Researchers have to keep in mind that reimbursements are different from incentives that are given to encourage people's involvement in studies. Incentives can become coercive. Significant incentives can persuade individuals to participate in the trial even if they are not interested. Besides these, recently, laws and regulations have been implemented for compensating research participants. Researchers have to be aware of the general rules related to compensation for research participation in the country before commencing clinical trials.

There should be a **grievance redressal** mechanism to address the participants' concerns. This mechanism can also be used to address participants' complaints that are unrelated to the intervention. Hence, a third-party body called a grievance redressal team should be present to address participant issues in real-time. Every trial has to have a pre-defined **trial stoppage** rule. As a rule of thumb, three pre-determined serious adverse events warrant the stoppage of a trial. These are death, serious complications of the previous clinical condition and hospitalisation due to any cause. If any of these three serious adverse events occur, an investigation has to be conducted to determine whether the adverse events are related to the trial. This investigation will be conducted by an independent third-party entity called Data Safety Monitoring Board. After scrutinising the adverse event, if the board permits, the trial can continue.

Documentation archival is another important point to be considered. The duration of document archival may differ among funding agencies, which may be five, 10 or even for 15 years. Investigators have to comply with the guidelines and regulations related to documentation archival of the funding agencies.

20.5 IMPEDIMENTS IN CLINICAL TRIAL PARTICIPATION

Patients may not be aware of or have access to clinical trials. Therefore, there is widespread mistrust as well as suspicion about trials. Thence, people are afraid to participate in them. Some people expect an exorbitant fee for participation that might not be affordable.

Patients or volunteers may not want to go against the advice of their healthcare providers. However, they must agree to participate voluntarily in the study. Hence, disseminating information on voluntary participation is essential. There are some issues **at the level of healthcare providers** as well. There is a lack of awareness among healthcare providers about clinical trials. Some healthcare providers may be unwilling to 'lose control' of their patients' care. There is fear among healthcare providers that they would lose their patients if they refer them for trials. They may also believe that standard therapy is the best. Further, they may be concerned about the administrative burdens associated with conducting trials.

Despite the impediments, quality-assured clinical trials are quintessential for making progress in medical science. If there are no clinical trials, no new drugs can be discovered, no new technologies can be implemented, and no new vaccines can be made available for the benefit of mankind. Hence, clinical trials must be supported, and adequate information about trials should be disseminated to participants and healthcare providers alike.

References and Further Reading

1. Poolman RW, Hanson B, Marti RK, Bhandari M. Conducting a clinical study: A guide for good research practice. Indian J Orthop 2007;41(1):27-31. https://www.ncbi.nlm.nih.gov/pmc/articles/PMC2981890/
2. Central Drugs Standards Control Organization (CDSCO). https://cdsco.gov.in/opencms/opencms/en/Home/
3. Chan AW, Tetzlaff JM, Gøtzsche PC, Altman DG, Howard M, Berlin JA et al. SPIRIT 2013 explanation and elaboration: guidance for protocols of clinical trials. BMJ 2013;346:e7586. https://www.bmj.com/content/bmj/346/bmj.e7586.full.pdf.

SECTION VI

WRITING A RESEARCH PROTOCOL

CHAPTER 21

PREPARING A CONCEPT PAPER FOR RESEARCH PROJECTS

P. Manickam

Learning Objectives

At the end of this chapter, readers will be able to:

1. Outline the elements of a concept paper
2. Translate a research idea into a one-page concept paper

So far, we have discussed the basics of research in terms of conceptualising the idea, choosing a study design, and ensuring ethical and scientific conduct of the research. This chapter will introduce you to preparing a concept paper for research projects.

21.1 STEPS OF EXECUTING A SUCCESSFUL PROTOCOL

There are seven logical, sequential and essential steps to executing a successful protocol. They are:

1. Identify the research topic and frame the research question and objectives
2. Outline a one-page concept paper
3. Prepare dummy tables and an analysis plan
4. Write a detailed draft protocol
5. Prepare study instruments and annexes
6. Submit the concept paper for peer review
7. Submit the concept paper for review by the ethics committee

Let's look at the life cycle of research. Research projects start with identifying data needs and ends with pointing out areas that require further investigation. A concept paper has to capture all of these elements in the miniature form of a protocol.

Rationale for Preparing a One-Page Concept Paper

Time is very precious for everybody—researchers, faculty, reviewers and even funders. A one-page concept note about the intended study will help save everybody's time and keep the researcher focused on the main goal of the research. Many of our ideas often remain as ideas and do not get transformed into research. Writing a one-page concept paper compared to a long and detailed protocol may help the researcher overcome the inhibition that they have to write a detailed protocol. Focusing on a single idea in a one-page concept paper will help the researcher convert the idea into action rather than getting aborted with a bunch of ideas alone.

21.2 OUTLINE OF A CONCEPT PAPER

A concept paper should have the following sequential sections in bulleted format.

1. Background and justification
2. Objectives
3. Methods
4. Expected benefits
5. References
6. Budget

21.2.1 Background and Justification

The background and justification for a research study can be explained by covering three points. First, the importance of the study problem; second, the known and unknown factors about the situation in literature and the local context; third, the information required to address the problem effectively. So, the first bullet should speak about the global consequences of the problem being studied, in terms of morbidity, mortality and effectiveness in the case of an intervention study. The second bullet should speak about the magnitude and influence of the health problem in the local context (state, district or local place of research). The third bullet should talk about the data needs of the study and describe the gaps in the currently available information.

21.2.2 Statement of Objectives

In a concept paper, not more than two or three objectives should be stated. The objectives may be split into 'general' and 'specific', if required. As discussed in the earlier chapters on research questions and goals, the purpose should be divided into primary and secondary objectives. This is critical because objectives clarify the reviewers about the research process.

21.2.3 Methods

The Methods section should provide information about the study design, study population, exposure and outcome variables, sample size calculation methodology and key considerations for sample size, sampling procedure and data collection, analysis plan, and human participant protection.

In the Methods section, the type of the study—whether it is a cross-sectional study, case-control study, cohort study or intervention study—should be stated and described. Then, details about the study population among whom the research will be conducted must be given, along with the eligibility criteria, the inclusion criteria and the exclusion criteria. In case of intervention studies, the randomisation and blinding procedures should be mentioned in this section. Then, the key operational definitions that will be used in the research need to be provided. The criteria for the operational definitions and participant selection strategies should also be mentioned. Then, the assumptions for sample size calculation, the calculated sample size and the sampling method using which the participants will be selected should be described briefly.

Additionally, the data collection procedure and quality assurance mechanism to be followed during data collection should be mentioned. Next, the primary outcomes of the research and the proposed plan of analysis should be described. Also, details of the type of analysis (descriptive, analytical, stratified or multivariate) and any additional research (such as subgroup analysis) should be provided. Finally, an explanation of how the researcher has addressed the ethical issues related to the protection of human participants must be given. The concept paper should state clearly whether an ethics review is needed for the research and if yes, which ethics committee will review the protocol.

21.2.4 Expected Benefits

Two aspects of benefits must be explained in answering the research question. One, what action will be taken following the results? Two, what is the future research, planning or policy plan resulting from these findings? These benefits must be explained in the concept paper. The concept paper should explicitly describe the expected outcome of the study and the timeline associated with it.

21.2.5 References

References can be provided in the Introduction section and operational definitions can be provided in the Methods section. You can add up to five references in your concept paper. We strongly recommend following internationally acceptable standard guidelines while writing these references. The globally accepted recommendation, the International Committee of Medical Journal Editors (ICMJE), should be adopted and used for referencing.

21.2.6 Budget

Budget is an equally important part in addition to the technical and other aspects of a concept paper. An indicative budget is sufficient at this stage; you need not provide a detailed justification for your intended expenses. Your budget can cover main items like salaries, per diem, transport costs, equipment costs, supplies and miscellaneous, and whatever other costs are applicable to conduct the research. Many research agencies insist on furnishing an indicative budget. Therefore, this is also an equally important part of a concept proposal.

21.3 APPLICATIONS OF CONCEPT PAPER

Let us look at some of the applications of a concept paper. The ICMR is a premier medical research agency that offers funds to researchers. To obtain this extramural funding, researchers must submit a pre-proposal or a concept proposal, similar to a concept paper. This concept proposal should have a title, introduction, novelty, applicability and description of the project. The ICMR suggests specific word count for each of these sections. Short-Term Studentship (STS) is another funding initiative of the ICMR, intended to support short projects pursued by medical undergraduates. The objective of this programme is to promote a research culture among medical undergraduates. An STS proposal must consist of a title, introduction, objective, methodology, implications and references. In this document, the Implications section is similar to the Expected Benefits section of the concept paper.

Many national and international agencies accept the pre-proposal, concept note or concept paper as a proof of concept for awarding funding for a research. This deliverable helps them screen the proposals for their worthiness and merit to earn the funds. Some research funding agencies even fund and support the development of a concept paper into a full-fledged protocol, if it is meritorious enough. Therefore, a well-designed and organised concept paper can help researchers source funding opportunities. The concept paper helps researchers organise their ideas and use the right words in a brief but concise manner to stand out among competition. A strong concept paper can help a researcher receive rapid and positive responses.

21.4 CONCEPT PAPER TEMPLATES

The template given in the appendix III will guide you in writing a concept paper. Here, we will discuss the templates of the concept paper for both observational and interventional studies.

21.4.1 Concept Paper for Observational Studies

In the appendix, you can find a template for an observational study design, covering the points discussed above. The first section of this concept paper covers the background and justification in three bullet points. The first bullet provides a context of the study problem in a quantified manner with linked references. The second bullet provides local context regarding what we know and what we do not know. The third bullet provides the information that we need to manage the problem effectively.

The next section provides the statement of objectives. Here, researchers should clarify whether they want to estimate a quantity or test a hypothesis, depending on the nature of the research question and statement of objectives. The primary objectives should be distinguished from the secondary objectives.

The following section covers the methods. The study design can be presented in one bullet in the Methods section. It could be a survey, case-control study, cohort study or ecological study, or sometimes even a case report or case series, depending on the study objectives. You can visit www.equator-network.org to access detailed reporting guidelines for different study designs that can be used to improve the reliability and quality of published health research literature. These guidelines can be followed while designing a study.

Following the study design, details about the eligible participants for the study who constitute the study population are given. The inclusion and exclusion criteria should be mentioned after the operational definitions, with references to the standard definition or criteria from the literature. Next, details about the sampling procedure, sample size, assumptions for calculating sample size and data collection procedure should be presented. The researcher should spell out who will collect the data, what kind of data will be collected, and within what time frame the data have to be collected. The quality assurance procedure for data collection should also be mentioned in this section. Additionally, a summarised plan for the analysis of data needs to be provided, based on the primary and secondary objectives. If there is a need for laboratory analysis, it should be documented along with its details.

Next, the researchers should explain the measures that are to be taken to ensure the protection of human participants. Then, the outcomes and benefits expected to be generated by the study should be described. The researcher may add up to five references for the study, according to the ICMJE guidelines. Finally, the budget should be explained in brief.

21.4.2 Concept Paper for Intervention Studies

For intervention studies, the concept paper should explain the background in terms of what is known and unknown about the drug or interventions or management of the specific research problem. The researchers need to explain why the available information is insufficient and state the objectives clearly, including the primary objective and how it will be reflected as the primary outcome. In the Methods section, the researcher can use the 'SPIRIT' guideline to write the clinical trial protocol. The Methods section of the concept paper is almost similar for observational and interventional studies, except for the fact that in an intervention or clinical trial concept paper, the interventions, the drug, its dosage, frequency, nature and additional interventions need to be specified. The primary and secondary outcomes should also be stated explicitly along with the operational definitions.

The next important section is on randomisation, sequence allocation and allocation concealment. The researchers must briefly mention the type and methods of randomisation that they will be using to generate and implement their selection of participants. They may also explain the participant recruitment strategy. Further, the level and description of masking should be mentioned. Apart from these, sample size assumptions and calculations need to be mentioned. The procedure for data collection and details of the analysis plan should also be described in the Methods section. The other sections, such as expected benefits, references and budget, are almost similar to the concept paper template for observational studies, which we have already discussed above.

A concept paper is a blueprint of your ideas. You can write a very good concept paper if you follow the templates given in the appendix for writing a concept paper.

References and Further Reading

1. Concept paper template for health research projects. ICMR School of Public Health, ICMR-National Institute of Epidemiology, Chennai, India. (Appendix III)

CHAPTER 22

ELEMENTS OF A PROTOCOL FOR RESEARCH STUDIES

Tarun Bhatnagar

Learning Objectives

At the end of this chapter, readers will be able to:

1. Describe the various steps in writing a research protocol
2. Outline the important components of a research

This chapter discusses the various elements of a research study protocol. The previous chapters explained how to design a research study, including how to decide on the research question, sampling, selecting study participants, measuring 'exposures' and 'outcomes' and ensuring human participant protection. All these fragments together form the structure of a research project. If the same is put down in a written format, it is called a 'protocol' or a written plan for a study.

22.1 SEVEN STEPS FOR WRITING A SUCCESSFUL PROTOCOL

The following are the steps for writing a successful protocol, as mentioned earlier in Chapter 21: Preparing a Concept Paper for Research Projects:

1. Identify the research topic, question and study objectives
2. Outline a one-page concept paper
3. Prepare dummy tables
4. Write a draft protocol
5. Prepare study instruments and annexes
6. Submit the concept paper for peer review
7. Seek ethics committee approval

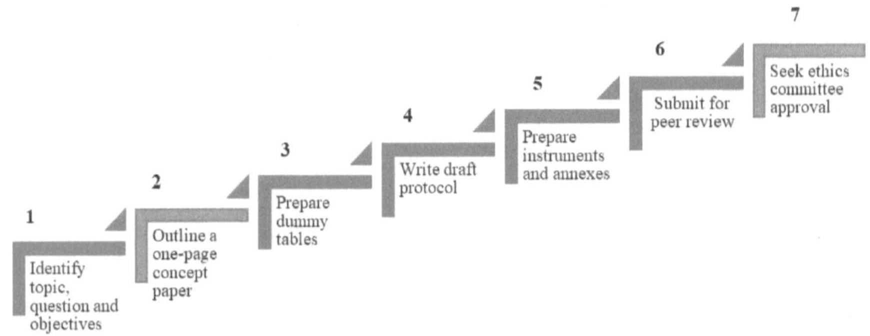

▲ **Figure 22.1:** Seven steps for developing a successful protocol

22.2 FIRST DRAFT OF THE PROTOCOL

The first draft of the research protocol can be written as soon as the researcher starts thinking about the topic of interest. Once the researcher drafts a concept paper, it can be used as an outline for developing the full-length protocol, describing in detail the points mentioned in the concept paper. The Objectives section of the protocol is retained as in the concept paper. The concept paper serves as a summary of the project protocol. The other elements such as background with justification, the method of conducting the study, expected benefits and budget that were briefly stated in the concept paper have to be detailed out in the protocol. The draft protocol should neither be too short nor too long. As a norm, the first draft should be written within 1500 to 2000 words and should not exceed 2000 words. The introduction should be focused and less than one-fifth of the total protocol. The draft protocol should contain at least five to ten key references. Further references can be added depending on the details that are added to the protocol.

22.3 OUTLINE OF THE METHODS SECTION

The Methods section is a significant part of the protocol that gives an idea about the detailed plan for conducting the study. In the Methods section, researchers have to elaborate on the appropriate study design, explain the interventions in experimental research, describe the study setting and study population, and spell out the operational definitions, method of sampling and method of sample size calculation. In addition, researchers must explain the data collection process and the tools used for it, the analysis plan, the project implementation plan with quality assurance and finally, the measures for human participant protection. Each of these components to be added in the Methods section is explained in the subsequent paragraphs to facilitate researchers in developing a protocol.

22.3.1 Study Design

Study design is the first sub-section under the Methods section. Here, researchers should explain how the objectives stated at the end of the Introduction section can be measured, how indicators can be framed to meet the objectives and what study design can be used to fulfil the stated objectives. The study design can be experimental or observational. If it is observational, it can be a cohort study, a case-control study or a cross-sectional study. The study design should be based on the objectives. Researchers should also mention whether the study will follow a 'prospective design' or a 'retrospective design', based on how one plans to collect data and how the particular investigation is designed.

22.3.2 Interventions

This sub-section describes the interventions, assuming that the researcher plans to conduct an experimental study. The intervention details should be provided both in clinical trials and community-based interventions. The details include:

- Who is going to face the intervention
- What exactly is the intervention—explained in detail
- What would be the period of intervention
- How would the intervention be done

This sub-section should also mention whether the researcher plans to conduct a clinical or community-based intervention.

22.3.3 Study Population

The inclusion and exclusion criteria for the study population should be stated explicitly. Inclusion and exclusion criteria describe the individual characteristics of the people the researcher intends to study or keep out of the study, respectively. Although the exclusion criteria can be added as a separate section, it does not differ conceptually from the inclusion criteria. This section should also state whether the study is hospital-based, community-based or population-based. Next, the researcher must mention the period for enrolling participants and conducting the survey. The geographical location of the participants and the characteristics of the participant group should also be mentioned. Remember that the study population is different from the study sample. The study population is the general population among whom one conducts the study. On the other hand, the study sample comprises the study participants who are chosen from the general population based on the sample size and sampling strategy employed. The researcher must ensure that the study population is suitable to address the objectives of the study.

22.3.4 Operational Definitions

In this sub-section, the researcher should provide workable definitions and how they intend to measure the key exposures and outcomes. The operational report must be clear and specific. If there are standard definitions and standard ways and means of measuring the variables, it is recommended to use them. In addition, the researcher should provide appropriate **references** for the description of variables and standard methods employed in the study.

22.3.5 Sampling Procedure

In this sub-section, the researcher should detail the sampling technique planned for the study. The types of sample used, such as random or non-random, convenience, systematic, cluster, etc., should be stated as applicable to the study. The details of how the researcher intends to select the study sample from the study population in practice have to be clearly stated in this sub-section. If the researcher intends to use standard sampling methods, it is prudent to provide references for the same as applied in other settings. In a randomised clinical trial, the researcher should explain how the randomisation would be done. The type of randomisation and the allocation of study participants for control and intervention groups should also be mentioned.

22.3.6 Sample Size

The sample size will depend on the study objective and the sampling methodology that the researcher intends to employ in the study. In this sub-section, the parameters to be used for the estimation should also be described. Also, details on whether the sample size was estimated using a software or formula and references for the parameters used in sample size estimation should be provided.

22.3.7 Data Collection

There are two parts to this sub-section. Firstly, the researcher should mention what information they plan to collect, such as social and demographic characteristics, individual characteristics of the study participants, clinical histories, which include signs and symptoms and so on. Secondly, the researcher should specify the exact way in which the data will be collected. Detailed information on who would be collecting the data and what data would be collected in the process has to be given. Here is an example: "The principal investigator or other investigators or trained data collectors or staff nurses or outreach workers will be collecting the data from the study participants". Next, details of how the data will be collected, such as the study instrument and the method of data collection, should be specified. In case of a quantitative research, the study instrument description should state whether data will be collected using a questionnaire or data abstraction form. For qualitative research, the study instrument description should provide the interview or topic guide with probes. For quantitative studies, a description of the method to be used for data collection, such as whether the data will be extracted by reviewing records or through one-to-one interviews or using a computer interface, should be given. Similarly, in case of a qualitative research, a description of methods such as whether focus group discussions or in-depth interviews will be employed should be given.

22.3.8 Analysis Plan

In this section, researchers should provide a detailed plan for data entry, data analysis and software use. They should state whether data entry would be done manually or using any software. If a software is to be used, its name should be mentioned. The details of re-categorisation and recoding can also be provided in this sub-section. The steps involved in analysing the collected data have to be laid down. Next, the manner in which the collected variables would be expressed, such as summary measures and statistical tests, should be stated. For example, in the case of descriptive studies, estimating prevalence or incidence, and in the case of analytical studies, whether it is univariate, stratified or multivariate analysis, keeping in mind the various steps and parameters.

Similarly, the researcher needs to describe the tests of significance that will be used to compare groups in the case of analytical studies and any other advanced statistical techniques, if any.

For example, a researcher conducts a cross-sectional study to examine the prevalence of

anaemia and associated factors among pregnant mothers in a district. The researcher plans to collect information on socio-demographic characteristics (such as age, education, occupation and income), clinical characteristics (such as haemoglobin level in gm/dl, birth order and pregnancy risk status), behavioural characteristics (such as tobacco consumption, hand hygiene and footwear usage) and obstetric information (such as trimester, number of hospital visits and number of iron and folic acid tablets consumed). The following is an excerpt of what the analysis section of this study may look like:

The data will be double-entered and validated using EpiData v.3.1 (Odense, Denmark). The data will then be exported to EpiAnalysis v. 2.2.3.187 for analysis. Variables such as age, income, haemoglobin level in gm/dl, birth order and number of hospital visits will be expressed as mean and standard deviation or median and interquartile range, depending on the normality of the distribution. Categorical variables such as occupation, risk status, tobacco consumption, hand hygiene, footwear usage and trimester will be expressed as numbers and proportions. Haemoglobin levels will be recorded as 'anaemia present' if the haemoglobin levels are less than 11gms/dl and 'anaemia absent' if the haemoglobin levels are equal to or more than 11gms/dl. The key analytic output, which is the prevalence of anaemia, will be expressed as number and proportion with a 95% confidence interval. To identify the factors associated with the presence of anaemia, first, an independent t-test or Mann-Whitney U test will be conducted for continuous variables such as age, income, birth order and the number of hospital visits with anaemia. A Chi-square test will be conducted for categorical variables such as occupation, risk status, tobacco consumption, hand hygiene, footwear usage and trimester with anaemia. Variables will be considered statistically significant if the p-value is less than 0.05. All variables with a p-value of less than 0.2 will be analysed using logistic regression. Unadjusted and adjusted prevalence ratio with a 95% confidence interval will be calculated to determine the presence of anaemia.

The analysis plan has to be clearly stated based on the study objectives. A vague statement stating that appropriate statistical analysis will be done would be inadequate. Such a statement will indicate that the researcher has not put in considerable efforts into the planning stage. Such an analysis plan will continue to remain unclear in the analysis stage.

22.3.9 Project Implementation Plan

This sub-section details the steps involved in implementing the study. A project implementation plan is a comprehensive quality assurance plan for data collection, data entry, data analysis and reporting of study results. This sub-section should also state the roles and responsibilities of the principal investigator, co-investigator and other workforce involved in the study, and the project governance—both administrative and technical. Details of how the project activities would be coordinated, the logistics of data collection in the field and the timeline should be specified here. The researcher has to mention the timeline for each phase of the study and the overall study period. The timeline should commence from the time taken for designing the instruments, getting approval from the ethics committee, pilot testing and actual data collection, followed by data entry, analysis, report writing and dissemination to the stakeholders until manuscript drafting and submission.

22.3.10 Human Participants' Protection

The last paragraph in the Methods section is on **human participants' protection.** Researchers should explain in detail the measures that they have taken to protect the study participants from any harm during or due to their participation in the study. This sub-section would include sub-headings such as **potential risks** that the participants may face during data collection and procedures that the researchers would employ to **minimise the risks,** emphasising **confidentiality** and **maximising the benefits** to the study participants. The sub-section should also include details of **compensations,** if any, without undue incentive, **informed consent**, whether oral or written, the personnel responsible for obtaining the consent, time taken to obtain consent, elements of consent and **approval procedures that a researcher would need** from the ethics committee of the institution.

22.3.11 Data Collection Instruments

Once all these elements in the protocol are put together, researchers should append the data collection instruments. Depending on the study design, study objectives and so forth, they should decide on the data collection instruments to be used in advance. In quantitative research, these may include **questionnaires, abstraction forms and a structured observation guide**. Similarly, an **interview guide for in-depth interviews** or a **topic guide for focus group discussions** can be used when employing qualitative methods. The study instruments should be translated into the local language that would be used for data collection. The study instrument must be available in both the language of the study and in the local language, based on the specific requirement.

22.4 ANNEXURES

Annexures should be placed at the end of the protocol. Annexures provide detailed information about the various components of the study implementation. These include forms for standard operating procedures, training framework for field workers, participant recruitment material, adverse event management forms, consent forms and study management forms. **Standard operating procedures** mention how the researchers collect data irrespective of the setting, whether it is field-based, laboratory-based or clinic-based. The **training framework** details how the researcher plans to train other investigators or field workers in collecting data. It also contains the training module for the same. The most important content to be added to the annexures is the **consent forms.** The annexures should contain the participant information sheet as well as the consent statement form, wherein the study participants sign, agreeing to participate in the study. As stated earlier, both these forms should be in English as well as the local language that would be used in the study.

22.5 FINALISING THE PROTOCOL

Writing a protocol is not a one-step process. It goes through several drafts before being finalised. It is wise to get the protocol **reviewed** by peers, who could be colleagues or subject experts. Based on their feedback, the researcher should revise and re-revise the protocol to get to a final stage when it can be submitted for **review** to the technical and ethics committees. These committees may suggest changes or revisions to the submitted protocol. Based on the suggestions, the researcher should again revise the protocol. Thus, the researcher would have multiple drafts of the protocol while arriving at the final version. It is a good practice to **archive all these drafts** so that the stakeholders know how the study evolved. Saving the drafts also helps to remember the different stages in which the study was planned.

22.6 RESOURCE MATERIAL

Reporting guidelines are available for specific study designs, such as observational studies, experimental studies, clinical trials, qualitative research, diagnostic studies, etc. There is also one for study protocols called "**SPIRIT** guidelines", which provides guidelines on writing a protocol for clinical trials. Other reporting guidelines include **CONSORT** for trials or **STROBE** for observation studies and **PRISMA** for meta-analysis and systematic reviews.

Although these are called reporting guidelines, a researcher can use these templates as a guide to draft their research protocols. Ultimately, the researcher's report should be based on the protocol.

22.7 LIFE CYCLE OF RESEARCH

Throughout this book, we have detailed the life cycle of research and examined the various steps involved in conducting a study. Following this life cycle is vital for conducting a focused and efficient analysis. When writing a study protocol or designing an investigation, researchers should make sure not to skip any of the steps of this life cycle. They should follow the procedure one step after another to draft a suitable protocol that is appropriate for the study objectives and the study design.

References and Further Reading

1. World Health Organization. Recommended format for a research protocol. WHO.https://www.who.int/ethics/review-committee/format-research-protocol/en/
2. Husain M. How to write a successful grant or fellowship application. PractNeurol 2015;15(6):474–8. https://pn.bmj.com/content/practneurol/15/6/474.full.pdf.

APPENDICES

The appendices can be downloaded from
https://nie.gov.in/icmr_sph/hrf-toolkit.html

APPENDIX I: SEQUENCE OF DATA ANALYSIS STRATEGY

1. **Identify study type**
   - Estimation or testing of hypothesis; review the study objectives

2. **Identify main variables**
   - Outcomes
   - Exposures
   - Potential confounders (a priori, before the analysis) (e.g., age, gender, socio-economic status….)
   - Variables for sub-group analysis

3. **Become familiar with the data**
   - Frequency distribution: Examine the frequency of all the variables
   - Descriptive statistics: All the variables describing the study population (See point 4 below).

4. **Characterize study population**
   - Demographic characteristics: Distribution of study participants (in case of an analytical study: for the two groups) by age, gender and so on
   - Clinical features: If applicable

5. **Examine outcome / exposure association on the basis of:**
   - Hypotheses: In case of an analytical study, compare the two groups for the frequency of exposures (See #2 above) using appropriate measure of association. Variables for which information was collected with multiple levels of exposure will be dichotomized a priori (before the analysis) on the basis of frequency distribution of exposure (e.g., median level of exposure).
   - Prior knowledge
   - Study design

6. **Create additional two-way tables (On the basis of analysis results)**
   - New variables: Spell out how you will create new variables (e.g., socio-economic score on the basis of few variables)
   - Decide whether you will require additional tables (e.g., results on the basis of weighted analysis; Results adjusted for age/gender)

7. **Conduct advanced analysis**
   - **Dose-response** (for variables associated with outcome in the univariate analysis, whether significant or not): Examine dose-response relationship by using the chi-square for trend (that can be examined with equal categories of exposures) or by using the regular chi-square (for variables for which the data was not available in equal categories of exposures).
   - **Stratified analysis:** Conduct stratified analysis to diagnose confounders or effect modifiers (i.e., that were associated with outcome in the univariate analysis)
   - **Multivariate analysis:** Determine the type of multivariate analysis required; Determine the variables to be included in the analysis [Outcome (independent) and Exposure (dependent or risk/protective factors); interaction terms]; conduct the multivariate analysis.

APPENDIX II: DUMMY TABLE SHELLS FOR REPORTS

Please cut and paste these tables into your own reports. After completion, apply checklist overleaf.

LIST OF TEMPLATE DUMMY TABLE SHELLS

PRACTICAL TIPS FOR THE PREPARATION OF DUMMY TABLE SHELLS BEFORE DATA ANALYSIS

1. Review the objectives of the study. Be clear about the study design that will be used (e.g., cohort versus or case control study) and about the indicators that will be calculated (e.g., relative risk or odds ratio).
2. List the full titles of all the tables to be prepared to meet the objectives (with time, place and persons characteristics). These titles may be written using the titles of the dummy tables as templates.
3. Identify the dummy tables from the list of "dummy tables for epidemiology reports" that can be used for the study at hand
4. Copy each dummy table needed under each title.
5. Modify the dummy table template to fit the study:
   a. Change column headings as required.
   b. Identify the broad groups of variables that the table will contain (e.g., demographic characteristics, education, income, occupation, family history, physical activity, tobacco use, obesity, diabetes status and co-morbidities) and place them as summary row headings.
   c. For each broad category of variables, identify the specific variables that will be used (e.g., Under "diabetes status", have "no diabetes", "pre-diabetes" and "diabetes").
   d. Dichotomize the variables of your study.
      - The plan should be to collect data in the field with multiple levels of exposure (e.g., mild, moderate, severe) or with quantitative data (e.g., exact monthly family income in rupees) to allow for the possibility to examine a dose-response relationship. However, to prepare a **summary** dummy table, anticipate a dichotomization that allows presenting a simple table that is easily readable.

- To dichotomize a variable, use any available biological rationale (e.g., CD4 cells < 200 denoting immuno-depression in the case of HIV infection) or the median of the frequency distribution (e.g., Monthly household income > median)

e. Avoid duplication of data (e.g., in the dummy table, for "sex", one line with "female sex" is sufficient as male sex can be deducted from the proportion of females).

f. Be specific about the variable to be mentioned in the dummy table. You must not only mention the variable, but also the value that it will take (e.g., Not "education", but "primary level"; Not "physical activity", but "moderate").

g. When preparing a dummy table for an analytical study, it helps to display factors that all go in the same direction (e.g., all risk factors for the disease, positively associated with the outcome: "low physical activity" and "tobacco use"). Note that this may require the use of negative in the dummy table (e.g., "low physical activity"). However, in the data collection instrument, it is better to collect data without using negative statements (e.g., the corresponding question should read "Do you exercise for at least 30 minutes daily?").

6. Use the checklists/guidelines/resources from the journals or standard guidelines (equator-network.org) for more resources

TABLE CHECKLIST

List of items	Explanation	Check (✓)
1. No fragmentation	Single table for data using same populations, denominators and indicators	☐
2. Alignment done	Numbers justified to the right hand side, text justified to the left hand side	☐
3. No calculation error	Totals and indicators checked for calculation errors (Use spreadsheet to develop table if possible)	☐
4. Rounding up	Proportions rounded at the percentage (no decimals) and measures of association rounded to 2 meaningful digits	☐
5. Clear headings	Short descriptive headings for rows and columns	☐
6. Complete title	Title describing the content of the cells of the table and providing time, place and person information	☐
7. Standardization	Dummy table template used	☐
8. Appropriate fonts	Use of capital letters limited to proper nouns and first letters of the table entries	☐
9. No acronyms	Use of acronyms limited to those standard (e.g., OR) explained by a footnote	☐
10. Footnotes	Additional details in footnotes, using standard caption symbols in the right order [Star (*), dagger (†), double-dagger (‡) etc…]	☐
11. Homogeneity of data	Homogeneous data in terms of populations, denominators and indicators (e.g., Don't mix means and proportions)	☐
12. Simplicity	Absence of redundant data	☐
13. Clarity of display	Landscape format, allowing sufficient space for descriptive row headings	☐
14. Ease of reading	One table per page	☐
15. Limited lines	Use of formatting lines limited to horizontal lines betweens sections of the table only	☐
16. Use of columns	Use of a separate column for each set of figures to ensure right alignment	☐
17. Data sorting	Rows sorted out (e.g., by increasing frequency) to facilitate accelerated reading	☐

▼ **Table 1:** Incidence of {disease} by age and sex, District, State, Country, Year

Demographic characteristics		Cases	20XX population	Incidence per 100,000
Age (years)	< 30	XXX	XX,XXX	XX
	30-45	XXX	XX,XXX	XX
	46-60	XXX	XX,XXX	XX
	>60	XXX	XX,XXX	XX
Gender	Male	XXX	XX,XXX	XX
	Female	XXX	XX,XXX	XX
Total		XXX	XX,XXX	XX

▼ **Table 2:** Descriptive characteristics of the study participants, District, State, Country, Year*

Characteristics		#	Total†	(%)
Age (Years)	< 30	XX	XX	XX
	30-45	XX	XX	XX
	46-60	XX	XX	XX
	>60	XX	XX	XX
Sex	Male	XX	XX	XX
	Female	XX	XX	XX
Education	Illiterate	XX	XX	XX
	Literate	XX	XX	XX
Socio-economic status‡	Below poverty line	XX	XX	XX
	Above poverty line	XX	XX	XX

* Use this dummy table for all descriptive characteristics (e.g., Characteristics of the cases, Prevalence of knowledge, attitude and practices)

† This column may be omitted if no missing values. In this case, indicate the number of cases (n=XX) in the title.

‡ As given by Niti Aayog

▼ **Table 3:** Frequency of selected exposures among {disease} cases and controls, case control study, District, State, Country, Year (Missing values)*

(Case scenario A: Total number of cases and controls vary because of missing values)

		Frequency of exposure †							
		Cases ‡			Controls §				
Characteristics		**#**	**Total**	**%**	**#**	**Total**	**%**	**Odds ratio**	**95% confi-dence interval**
Demographic characteristics	**Age > median age**	XX	XX	XX	XX	XX	XX	X.X	X.X-X.X
	Female sex	XX	XX	XX	XX	XX	XX	X.X	X.X-X.X
Risk factors	**Obesity**	XX	XX	XX	XX	XX	XX	X.X	X.X-X.X
	Family history	XX	XX	XX	XX	XX	XX	X.X	X.X-X.X
	Tobacco use	XX	XX	XX	XX	XX	XX	X.X	X.X-X.X
	Absence of physical activity	XX	XX	XX	XX	XX	XX	X.X	X.X-X.X
	Co-morbidities	XX	XX	XX	XX	XX	XX	X.X	X.X-X.X

* First footnote is a star

† Second footnote is a dagger

‡ Third footnote is a double dagger

§ Fourth footnote is a paragraph sign

▼ **Table 4:** Frequency of selected exposures among {disease} cases and controls, case control study, District, State, Country, Year (No missing values)

(Case scenario B: Total number of cases and controls identical in the absence of missing values)

		Frequency of exposure					
		Cases (n=XX)		Controls (n=XX)			
Characteristics		#*	%	#*	%	Odds ratio	95% confidence interval
Demographic characteristics	**Age > median age**	XX	XX	XX	XX	X.X	X.X-X.X
	Female sex	XX	XX	XX	XX	X.X	X.X-X.X
Risk factors	**Obesity**	XX	XX	XX	XX	X.X	X.X-X.X
	Family history	XX	XX	XX	XX	X.X	X.X-X.X
	Tobacco use	XX	XX	XX	XX	X.X	X.X-X.X
	Absence of physical activity	XX	XX	XX	XX	X.X	X.X-X.X
	Co-morbidities	XX	XX	XX	XX	X.X	X.X-X.X

* In a slide set for an oral presentation, this column may be omitted to simplify.

▼ **Table 5:** Incidence of {disease} according to selected characteristics, cohort study, District, State, Country, Year*

Characteristics		Incidence of disease: Among exposed #	Among exposed Total	Among exposed %	Among unexposed #	Among unexposed Total	Among unexposed %	Relative risk	95% confidence interval
Demographic characteristics	**Age > median age**	XX	XX	XX	XX	XX	XX	X.X	X.X-X.X
	Female sex	XX	XX	XX	XX	XX	XX	X.X	X.X-X.X
Risk factors	**Obesity**	XX	XX	XX	XX	XX	XX	X.X	X.X-X.X
	Family history	XX	XX	XX	XX	XX	XX	X.X	X.X-X.X
	Tobacco use	XX	XX	XX	XX	XX	XX	X.X	X.X-X.X
	Absence of physical activity	XX	XX	XX	XX	XX	XX	X.X	X.X-X.X
	Co-morbidities	XX	XX	XX	XX	XX	XX	X.X	X.X-X.X

* This table can be adopted for intervention studies; Replace incidence of disease among exposed and unexposed by incidence of primary outcome among intervention groups

▼ **Table 6:** Prevalence of {disease} according to selected characteristics, cross sectional study, District, State, Country, Year

		Prevalence of disease							
		Among exposed			Among unexposed				
Characteristics		**#**	**Total**	**%**	**#**	**Total**	**%**	**Prevalence ratio**	**95% confidence interval**
Demographic	**Age > median age**	XX	XX	XX	XX	XX	XX	X.X	X.X-X.X
Characteristics	**Female sex**	XX	XX	XX	XX	XX	XX	X.X	X.X-X.X
	Obesity	XX	XX	XX	XX	XX	XX	X.X	X.X-X.X
	Family history	XX	XX	XX	XX	XX	XX	X.X	X.X-X.X
Risk factors	**Tobacco use**	XX	XX	XX	XX	XX	XX	X.X	X.X-X.X
	Absence of physical activity	XX	XX	XX	XX	XX	XX	X.X	X.X-X.X
	Co-morbidities	XX	XX	XX	XX	XX	XX	X.X	X.X-X.X

▼ **Table 7:** Frequency of selected exposures among those with and without the prevalence of the condition, cross-sectional study, District, State, Country, Year (No missing values)

		Frequency of exposure					
		Present (n=XX)		Absent (n=XX)			
Characteristics		**#***	**%**	**#***	**%**	**Prevalence odds ratio**	**95% confidence interval**
Demographic	**Age > median age**	XX	XX	XX	XX	X.X	X.X-X.X
characteristics	**Female sex**	XX	XX	XX	XX	X.X	X.X-X.X
	Obesity	XX	XX	XX	XX	X.X	X.X-X.X
	Family history	XX	XX	XX	XX	X.X	X.X-X.X
Risk factors	**Tobacco use**	XX	XX	XX	XX	X.X	X.X-X.X
	Absence of physical activity	XX	XX	XX	XX	X.X	X.X-X.X
	Co-morbidities	XX	XX	XX	XX	X.X	X.X-X.X

* In a slide set for an oral presentation, this column may be omitted to simplify.

▼ **Table 8:** Distribution of {disease} case control sets according to the exposure status of the cases and control, District, State, Country, Year*

		Number of case control sets					
		Concordant for exposure status		Discordant for exposure status			
		Case exposed	Case unexposed	Case exposed	Case unexposed	Odds ratio	95% confidence interval
Socio-economic Status	Monthly income > median	XX	XX	XX	XX	X.X	X.X-X.X
	Primary education	XX	XX	XX	XX	X.X	X.X-X.X
Risk factors	Obesity	XX	XX	XX	XX	X.X	X.X-X.X
	Family history	XX	XX	XX	XX	X.X	X.X-X.X
	Tobacco use	XX	XX	XX	XX	X.X	X.X-X.X
	Absence of physical activity	XX	XX	XX	XX	X.X	X.X-X.X
	Co-morbidities	XX	XX	XX	XX	X.X	X.X-X.X

* Assuming matching for age and sex, therefore these variables are not in the table.

▼ **Table 9:** Distribution of matched case control sets according to the exposure of the cases and the two controls. District, State, Country, Year

Status of the case	Number of controls exposed	Number of discordant pairs in the set		Number of sets in the category		Total number of discordant pairs in the category	Total number of discordant pairs*
Exposed	2 controls exposed	X	x	X	=	XX	XX (f)
	1 control exposed, 1 unexposed	X	x	X	=	XX	
	0 control exposed	X	x	X	=	XX	
Unexposed	2 controls exposed	X	x	X	=	XX	XX (g)
	1 control exposed, 1 unexposed	X	x	X	=	XX	
	0 control exposed	X	x	X	=	XX	

▼ **Table 10:** Odds of {disease} according to increasing gradients of {exposure}, District, State, Country, Year

Exposure	Cases (n=XX)		Controls (n=XX)		Odds ratio	95% CI
	#	%	#	%		
Level 0	XX	XX	XX	XX	1 (Reference)	-
Level 1	XX	XX	XX	XX	X.X	X.X-X.X
Level 2	XX	XX	XX	XX	X.X	X.X-X.X
Level 3	XX	XX	XX	XX	X.X	X.X-X.X
Level 4	XX	XX	XX	XX	X.X	X.X-X.X

* Matched odds ratio = f / g = XX

▼ **Table 11:** Factors associated with {disease} in multiple logistic regression, District, State, Country, Year

Characteristics	Crude odds ratio	Adjusted odds ratio	
		Estimate*	95% confidence interval
Low physical activity	X.X	X.X	X.X-X.X
Moderate physical activity	X.X	X.X	X.X-X.X
Obesity (BMI>25)	X.X	X.X	X.X-X.X
Family history (One or more blood relative with a known history of type 2 diabetes)	X.X	X.X	X.X-X.X

* No physical activity, normal BMI and no family history were taken as reference categories

APPENDIX III: CONCEPT PAPER FOR – [INSERT TITLE OF THE PROJECT HERE]

Insert name of primary investigator here

Background - justification
• Review in a first bullet the global public health consequences of the problem being examined in terms of death, disability, effectiveness and cost-effectiveness of interventions. Avoid general statements and provide quantified data when available. Follow by explaining how this problem affects the region where the project is being considered. • Provide information on completed, ongoing or planned prevention and control efforts targeting this problem in South Asia, India and / or the state where the project will be conducted. • Specify (1) the data that are needed by the prevention and control programme to improve this public health problem and (2) why the data currently available are not sufficient.
Objectives
• Spell out first objective. Make sure that you make it clear whether you propose to *estimate a quantity* (e.g., prevalence, incidence) or whether you propose to *test a hypothesis.* • Spell out second objective. Make sure that you make it clear whether you propose to *estimate a quantity* (e.g., prevalence, incidence) or whether you propose to *test a hypothesis.* • Spell out third objective. Make sure that you make it clear whether you propose to *estimate a quantity* (e.g., prevalence, incidence) or whether you propose to *test a hypothesis.*
Proposed methods
Study population • Specify the population in which you will undertake the study (State, district, population size.) **Study design** • Describe the type of study (e.g., survey, case-control study) in one short bullet **Operational Definitions** • Provide information regarding the key case definitions, criteria and / or control recruitment strategy that you will be using. **Sampling procedure** • Describe the type of sampling you will be using **Sample size** • Briefly mention your sample size and the main assumptions you used to calculate it. This should contain enough information for the reader to redo the calculations to check the estimate. **Data collection** • Explain shortly who will collect what kind of data, what the timeline is and what quality assurance mechanism will be used. **Analysis plan** • Summarize the type of analysis (e.g., descriptive, analytical, stratified, multivariate) that you plan to carry out. Mention laboratory analysis if they will be part of the study. **Human participant protection** • Mention key measures taken to ensure the protection of human participants in your study and whether ethical committee review will be needed, expedited, or not needed (exempt).

Expected benefit
• Describe the expected output (e.g., reports) that this study will generate and the timeline. • Describe the expected outcome: How this study will influence prevention and control activities for the problem in question in the area where the project will be conducted.
Budget
• Staff (Salary and per diem): Rs. XXXXX • Transport: Rs. XXXXX • Supplies (e.g., laboratory reagents, stationery, and others): Rs. XXXX • Miscellaneous: Rs. XXXXX **Total amount needed: Rs. XXXXXX**

ABOUT THE AUTHORS

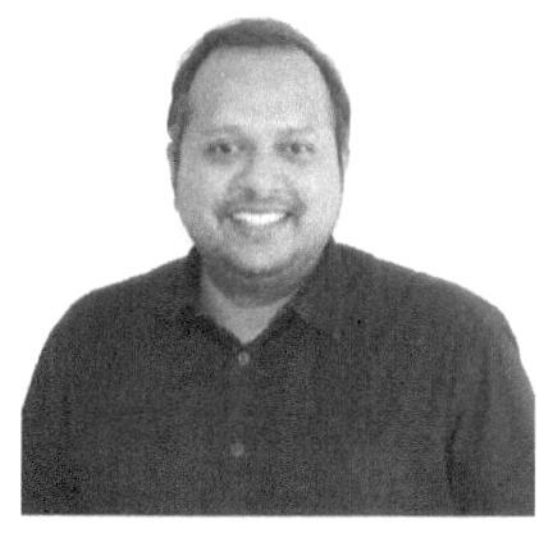

Dr. P. Ganesh Kumar, MBBS, MD
(Community Medicine)
Scientist D, ICMR-National Institute of Epidemiology

Dr P. Ganesh Kumar serves as Scientist-D (Medical) at ICMR-NIE. He did Doctorate of Medicine in Community Medicine. He serves as course coordinator and core faculty for Field epidemiology training programs at ICMR NIE since 2014. He is currently working under the Division of Epidemiology at ICMR-NIE. His research areas include (a) Health Systems Research (b) Digital health (c) Public health surveillance (d) Noncommunicable diseases. He has co-authored over 50 publications.

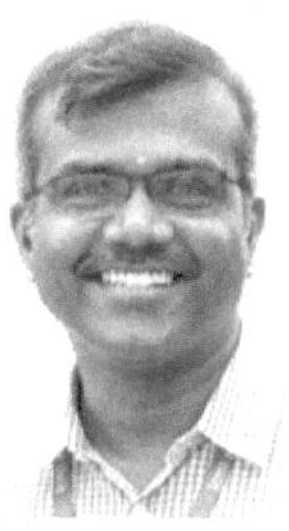

Dr. P. Manickam, BSMS, MSc (Epid), PhD
Scientist F, ICMR-National Institute of Epidemiology

P. Manickam serves as Scientist F (Epidemiology) at the ICMR-NIE. He is a trained physician in Siddha System of Medicine, one of India's Ayush systems based in South India. He did Masters and Ph.D., in Epidemiology and advanced studies health district management. He heads the Division of Online Courses and responsible for the Institute's initiative on Massive Open Online Courses (MOOCs) in health research. He serves as core faculty member for two-year Master's level public health training program of ICMR School of Public Health at ICMR-NIE since 2001. He guides doctoral program in epidemiology and teaches in several short-term courses since 2001. His focus areas are capacity building in public health, outbreak science, surveillance and response to public health emergencies & during mass gatherings and clinical research in traditional medicine. He has published 100 manuscripts in biomedical journals and three chapters in books.

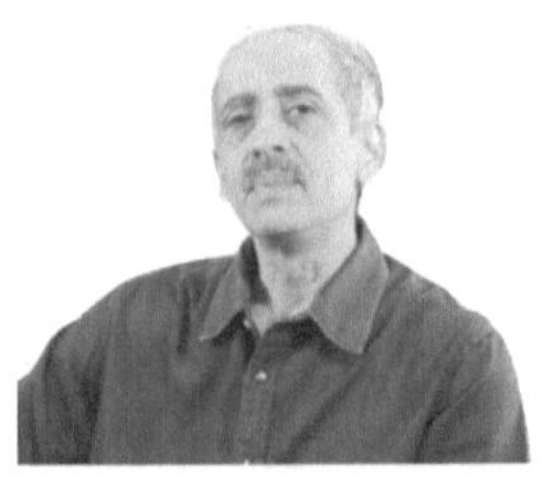

Dr. Manoj V Murhekar, MBBS, MD
(Preventive and Social Medicine)
Scientist G & Director, ICMR-National Institute of Epidemiology

Dr Murhekar is currently the Director and Scientist-G at the ICMR-National Institute of Epidemiology (NIE), Chennai, a permanent institute of the Indian Council of Medical Research. He obtained his MBBS and MD in community medicine from Government Medical College, Nagpur, Maharashtra, India. His research interests include Infectious disease epidemiology, vaccine-preventable diseases, and disease surveillance and outbreak investigations. He is also the course director for the field epidemiology training program (FETP) that ICMR-NIE is conducting since 2001.

Prior to joining ICMR-NIE, Dr Murhekar worked at the ICMR-Regional Medical Research Centre in Port Blair on the Andaman and Nicobar Islands. He was awarded the Major General Saheb Singh Sokhey Award of the Indian Council of Medical Research for his contribution to the field of viral hepatitis among the tribal population of Andaman and Nicobar. He has about 300 publications in peer-reviewed journals to his credit. He is the associate editor of the journal BMC Infectious Diseases

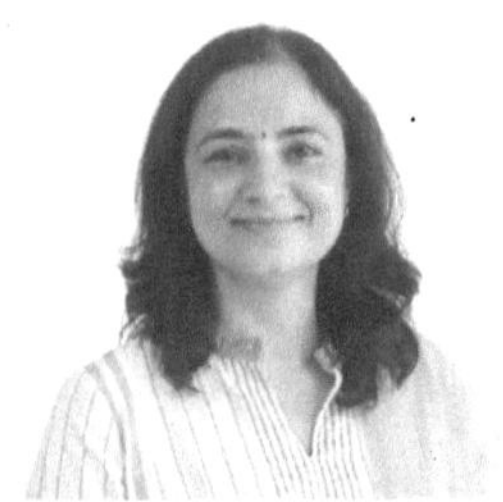

Dr Prabhdeep Kaur, DNB (General Medicine), MAE (FETP)
Professor, Issac Centre for Public Health, Indian Institute of Science
Former Scientist F, ICMR-National Institute of Epidemiology

Dr Prabhdeep Kaur is a physician and public health professional, currently working as a Professor at the Issac Centre for Public Health, Indian Institute of Science, Bengaluru. She was a former Scientist F and Head of Division of Noncommunicable Diseases and Course Coordinator for the FETP Fellowships (Advanced 2 year and Intermediate 1 year) at ICMR-National Institute of Epidemiology, Chennai. She did her post-graduation in Internal medicine and Masters Applied Epidemiology in India and has 19 years of experience in epidemiological research, teaching, and implementation science. She worked in a wide range of areas, including public health initiatives to improve the prevention and treatment of hypertension, diabetes and cervical cancer and epidemiological research for various NCDs. She is the Principal Investigator for the "India Hypertension Control Initiative", a multi-partner implementation science project implemented in 130+ districts across 23 states to improve hypertension treatment and control. She was a member of the Chief Minister's Expert Task Force for COVID-19 control in Tamil Nadu, India, 2020-21. She provided technical support to Govt. of Punjab for the first pilot project to introduce the HPV vaccine in India. She is a member of the WHO's Global Cervical Cancer Elimination Expert group (2019-2022). She led various multisite projects, notably the Concurrent evaluation of the NCD program under the Tamil Nadu Health Systems Project in 32 districts (2008-15), NCD mortality among tribal populations, and health systems preparedness in 12 states (2015-18). The scientific work led to 80+ papers in national/ international peer-reviewed journals.

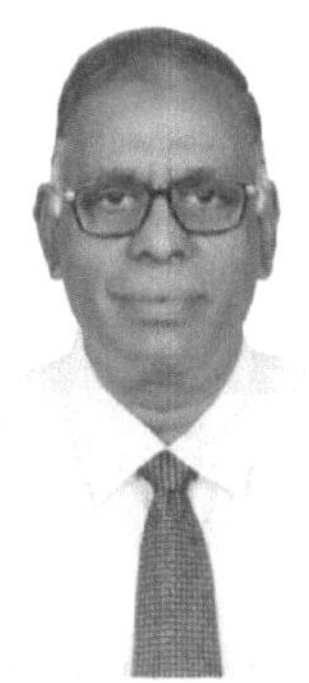

Dr.R. Ramakrishnan, M.Sc.,Ph.D.,M.A.E
Scientist G(Retd.), ICMR-National Institute of Epidemiology,

R. Ramakrishnan superannuated from ICMR-NIE as Scientist G in 2016. He served as Consultant, DHR for two years and as the visiting faculty at the Central University of Tamil Nadu (CUTN) for two years. He has a PhD in Statistics from the University of Madras and a Masters in Applied Epidemiology (MAE) from the Australian National University. He carried out several National/ International collaborative projects in various fields – Communicable diseases, Health Systems Research and methodological studies. He has more than 50 publications. He was one of the core faculties at the ICMR School of Public Health, NIE. Presently, he is serving as Chairman/ Member of several Institutional Ethics Committee and Review Board.

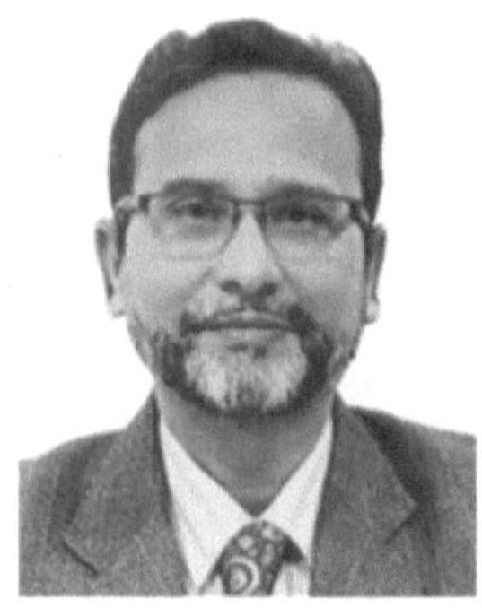

Dr. Sanjay Mehendale, MD, MPH, FACE, FIMSA, FAMS

Director of Research, PD Hinduja National Hospital and Medical Research Center

Former Additional Director General, Indian Council of Medical Research [ICMR]

Former Director, ICMR-National Institute of Epidemiology

Dr. Mehendale's total research career covers 6 years in BJ Medical College, Pune, 32 years in Indian Council of Medical Research and 4 years at Hinduja Hospital, Mumbai. He started his career in ICMR at ICMR - National Institute of Virology, in Pune where he conducted many field-based studies related to dengue fever, Japanese encephalitis, hepatitis, measles, and hemorrhagic fevers. Dr. Mehendale led several sero-epidemiological studies, clinical trials and socio-behavioral studies related to HIV/ AIDS during his research tenure at ICMR – National AIDS Research Institute. Dr. Mehendale then served as Director of ICMR - National Institute of Epidemiology, in Chennai from 2010 to 2016. Under his leadership, MSc program in Biostatistics affiliated to Periyar University and an online course "Health Research Fundamentals" by National Institute of Epidemiology were launched. In September 2016, Dr. Mehendale assumed the charge of Additional Director General of the Indian Council of Medical Research, Department of Health Research, Govt. of India, New Delhi until his superannuation in 2018. Dr. Sanjay Mehendale is currently working as Director Research at PD Hinduja Hospital and Medical Research Center in Mumbai. Dr. Mehendale has served as Chairperson as well as Member of several scientific committees, expert committees and ethics committees. He has conducted several training courses on research methodology, bioethics, and clinical trials, and has published more than 210 research papers in national and international journals and 9 book chapters.

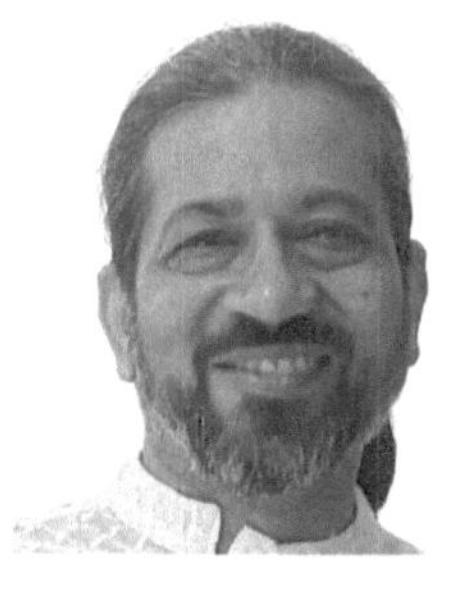

Dr. Tarun Bhatnagar, MD (PSM), PhD (Epid), PGDBE

Scientist F, ICMR-National Institute of Epidemiology Chennai, India

Dr. Tarun Bhatnagar, MD (Preventive & Social Medicine) from Banaras Hindu University, Varanasi, India, PhD (Epidemiology) from University of California, Los Angeles, USA, and Postgraduate Diploma in Bioethics from Indira Gandhi National Open University, India currently works in the position of Scientist-F and Head, ICMR School of Public Health at the ICMR–National Institute of Epidemiology in Chennai, India. His research interests include epidemiological methods, causality, HIV prevention research, epidemiology of emerging infectious disease (Nipah virus, Zika virus, COVID-19), cohort studies, health systems research, and evaluation of public health control strategies/programs. Dr. Bhatnagar has authored 80+ research publications in scientific journals and 4 book chapters.

www.ingramcontent.com/pod-product-compliance
Lightning Source LLC
LaVergne TN
LVHW041155150826
845673LV00001B/171

* 9 7 9 8 8 8 9 3 5 9 4 1 8 *